Practical Vascular Ultrasound

An Illustrated Guide

Practical
Vascular
Ultrasound

An
Illustrated
Guide

Kenneth Myers - MS FRACS FACS DDU(Vasc)
Consultant Vascular Surgeon, Monash Medical Centre, and Consultant in Vascular Imaging,
Victoria Vascular Ultrasound, Melbourne, Victoria, Australia.

Amy May Clough - BSc DMU (Vasc) AMS
Senior Vascular Ultrasonographer, Victoria Vascular Ultrasound, Melbourne, Victoria, Australia

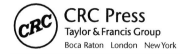

CRC Press
Taylor & Francis Group
Boca Raton   London   New York

CRC Press is an imprint of the
Taylor & Francis Group, an informa business

CRC Press
Taylor & Francis Group
6000 Broken Sound Parkway NW, Suite 300
Boca Raton, FL 33487-2742

© 2014 by Taylor & Francis Group, LLC
CRC Press is an imprint of Taylor & Francis Group, an Informa business

No claim to original U.S. Government works

Printed on acid-free paper
Version Date: 20140213

International Standard Book Number-13: 978-1-4441-8118-0 (Paperback)

Library of Congress Cataloging-in-Publication Data

Myers, Kenneth A. (Surgeon), author.
  Practical vascular ultrasound : an illustrated guide / Kenneth Myers, Amy May Clough.
  p. ; cm.
  Includes bibliographical references and index.
  ISBN 978-1-4441-8118-0 (pbk. : alk. paper)
  I. Clough, Amy, author. II. Title.
  [DNLM: 1. Vascular Diseases--ultrasonography. 2. Blood Vessels--anatomy & histology. 3. Ultrasonography,
Doppler. 4. Ultrasonography, Interventional. 5. Vascular Diseases--surgery. WG 500]

  RC691.6.U47
  616.1'307543--dc23   2014004760

**Visit the Taylor & Francis Web site at
http://www.taylorandfrancis.com**

**and the CRC Press Web site at
http://www.crcpress.com**

Contents

Preface

As technology for vascular ultrasound continues to rapidly evolve, it has become more than just an adjunct to other imaging modalities but provides a firm basis for deciding the most appropriate interventional treatment for vascular disease. This is especially true for venous ultrasound, which we believe is now the "gold standard". However, unlike other imaging modalities, ultrasound is highly subjective and relies on Sonographers and Sonologists with well developed expertise and thorough knowledge of machine optimisation as well as vascular anatomy, physiology and pathology.

Practical Vascular Ultrasound provides imperative background information for relevant physiology and pathology and general principles of vascular scanning. The book ultimately aims to concisely but comprehensively present basic anatomy and clinical aspects, and to extensively describe scanning protocols and criteria for each anatomical region of interest. The book also covers use of ultrasound for guiding vascular procedures.

Practical Vascular Ultrasound is designed to be a hands-on book for rapid reference in the course of day-to-day practice. We feel that it provides an easy to understand guide for those who are learning the art and indeed for experienced practitioners who wish to touch up their skills. *Practical Vascular Ultrasound* has been written with the aim to achieve a consistent, comprehensive and professional approach to vascular ultrasound.

Kenneth Myers
Amy May Clough

Foreword

This is the much awaited revision of the well-known *Making Sense of Vascular Ultrasound*. There have been many changes which enhance its breadth of information. As before, the presentation has great clarity.

It again has the appropriate balance between clinical aspects based on anatomy and pathology leading to a logical approach to applying these to normal vascular ultrasound findings and ultrasound manifestations of vascular disease. Throughout, there is a balanced approach to the selection of ultrasound or other imaging modalities.

After chapters that deal with basic anatomy and pathology as well as application of ultrasound principles to vascular studies, the book then covers every accessible area of the body for both arterial and venous studies, with welcome additions to studies for vascular tumours and malformations, hemodialysis and male genital vascular disorders.

Each chapter is comprehensive and concise with excellent illustrations that enhance the clarity of presentation. As well as developing optimal techniques and interpretation, each regional chapter indicates what referring doctors need to know and hints and tips as well as pitfalls and warnings, while most chapters have representative simple worksheets that the authors have developed in their practice.

The book is based on past experience gained by the authors over many years. Indeed, I have been fortunate to collaborate and work with the authors virtually since the clinical introduction of vascular ultrasound. The book is highly recommended to all trainee and practising vascular ultrasonographers, vascular surgeons and internists and vascular researchers.

Andrew Nicolaides

Acknowledgments

Ken Myers

To Andrew Nicolaides and Alan Bray who introduced me to Vascular ultrasound.

To my practice partner, Dr Stefania Roberts, for her help and for putting up with this enterprise that so disrupted our practice at times. Also to my other medical colleagues, Dr Martine Apikian and Dr Sharon Felzen for their support. To the rest of our team, Janet Hargreaves, Jacqui Kirwan, Nicole Hendriks and Antoinette Natoli with thanks.

Amy May Clough

To my darling sister – Bec Clough.

To my friends – Katie Wittman, Erica McCalman, Erik Rau, Gareth Larson, Hollie Perniskie and Claire Gibbs for your support and laughter.

Much gratitude to my colleagues - Martine Apikian, Antoinette Natoli, Stef Roberts, Janet Hargreaves, Jax Kirwan, Sharon Felzen and Nicole Hendriks.

Special thank you to Martin Necas for your light heartedness and professional support.

VASCULAR PHYSIOLOGY

Understanding pulsatile flow in compliant blood vessels is more complex than applying physical laws relating to steady flow in rigid tubes, but the latter provide a guide.

BLOOD FLOW IN ARTERIES

Symbols used and abbreviations with units in brackets:

- A – cross-sectional area (cm^2)
- C – compliance (1/Pa)
- CO – cardiac output (ml)
- CVP – central venous pressure (mmHg)
- d – diameter (cm)
- D – shear rate (/s)
- g – acceleration due to gravity = 980 cm/s^2
- h – height (cm)
- l – length (cm)
- MAP – mean arterial pressure (mmHg)
- N – number of branches
- P – pressure (1 mmHg = 1333 dyn/cm^2)
- PSV – peak systolic velocity (cm/s)
- Δp – pulse pressure at one site (systolic − diastolic pressure)
- ΔP – pressure gradient between two sites or perfusion pressure
- Q – flow (ml/s)
- r – internal radius (cm)
- r_1 – diameter in a proximal arterial segment relatively free from disease
- r_2 – diameter at the stenosis
- Δr – change in radius with the pulse (mm)
- R – resistance (dyn s/cm)
- R' – single vessel resistance (dyn s/cm)
- Re – Reynolds' number for turbulence (dimensionless)
- t – arterial wall thickness (mm)
- T – shear stress (dyn/cm^2)
- TPR – total peripheral resistance (dyn s/cm)
- v – velocity (cm/s)
- Δv – change in velocity (cm/s)
- ρ – fluid density (g/cm^3) = 1.056 for blood
- η – coefficient of viscosity (poise).

Blood pressure

- Blood pressure is the force per unit area exerted by blood on the vessel wall.
- Pressure in an elastic tube is determined by:
  - Volume of fluid in the tube.
  - Compliance of the tube wall.

- Arteries are thick walled and not very compliant. They contain approximately 10% of blood volume at a mean pressure of approximately 100 mmHg.
- Veins are thin walled and compliant. They contain approximately 60% of blood volume at a pressure of <10 mmHg:

$$C = \Delta v / \Delta P$$

- Blood pressure regulation is determined by:

$$MAP = CO \times TPR$$

Where MAP is the average of the arterial pressure over one heart cycle, CO is the volume of blood ejected by the left ventricle into the aorta within a minute, and TPR is the net flow resistance in the systemic loop.

Flow rate, flow velocity, and blood flow

- The human circulation is a closed system of tubes.
- The flow rate is the total volume of blood that passes a given point in a vessel per unit time.
- The flow rate through an artery or the sum of its branches averaged over time is constant.
- This is expressed as the *continuity equation of flow*:

$$Q = vA \text{ or } v = Q/A = Q/\pi r^2$$

- Using this equation, a 50% diameter reduction in an artery should increase velocity by four times but it is less than this in the circulation.
- Blood flow is proportional to the blood pressure gradient.
- The driving force for blood to flow is due to the difference in MAP and CVP in the form of a pressure gradient.
- It is defined by a derivation of *Ohm's law*:*

$$Q = MAP - CVP/TPR$$

or

$$Q = \Delta P/TPR$$

- Direction of flow is from high to low pressure.
- TPR has more influence on blood pressure than perfusion pressure.
- Blood also flows in arteries due to left ventricular contraction pressures (force per unit area).

Energy for blood flow

- Physical principles relating to ideal fluid motion in hollow tubes assume that the flow velocity is constant, the flow is smooth with no turbulence, the tube is straight, rigid, and with no branches, and the fluid is non-viscous and incompressible.
- The driving pressure for flow is determined by its potential energy (PE) and its kinetic energy (KE).
- *PE* is the latent capacity to do work and results in considerable pressure variations when standing (Fig. 1.1). PE is determined by fluid density, acceleration due to gravity, and height of the column:

$$PE = \rho g h$$

- PE can be expressed as the 'hydrostatic head of pressure'.

---

*Georg Simon Ohm, 1789–1854, German physicist

- *KE* is the energy resulting from the fluid flow and increases where a tube narrows (Fig. 1.2). KE is determined from fluid density and velocity:

$$KE = \tfrac{1}{2}\rho v^2$$

- Conservation of energy requires that pressures at two points (1 and 2) along a tube are ideally expressed as *Bernoulli's equation*:*

$$P_1 + \rho gh_1 + \tfrac{1}{2}\rho v_1^2 = P_2 + \rho gh_2 + \tfrac{1}{2}\rho v_2^2$$

or

$$\Delta P = \rho g(h_2 - h_1) + \tfrac{1}{2}\rho(v_2^2 - v_1^2)$$

- An important consequence of Bernoulli's equation is the conservation of PE as KE or an increase in blood pressure, and an increase in velocity results in a decrease in pressure.

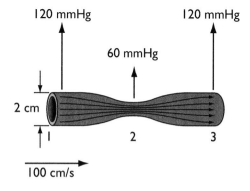

Arterial pressure (mmHg)	Height (cm)	Venous pressure (mmHg)
120 – 50 = 70	60	0
120 + 0 = 120	0	10 + 0 = 10
120 + 80 = 200	–100	10 + 80 = 90

Fig. 1.1 *Potential energy.*
- *Fluid flows from a low pressure (high PE) at the heart to a high pressure (low PE) at the feet.*
- *If h = 100 cm from heart to feet while standing, then:*

$$\Delta P = \rho g(h_2 - h_1)$$

$$= 1.056 \times 980 \times 100$$

$$= 103,488 \text{ dyn/cm}^2$$

$$\approx 80 \text{ mmHg}$$

120 mmHg   120 mmHg

60 mmHg

2 cm

↑1   2   3

100 cm/s

Low velocity
Low KE
High pressure

High velocity
High KE
Low pressure
Streamlines closer

Low velocity
Low KE
High pressure

Fig. 1.2 *Kinetic energy.*
- *Fluid flows from a low to a high KE region at a narrowing to cause substantial pressure drop.*
- *If the inlet (1) has a diameter of 2 cm, fluid is flowing at 100 cm/s and diameter at a narrowing (2) is 1 cm, so that velocity theoretically increases to 400 cm/s, then:*

$$\Delta P = \tfrac{1}{2}\rho(v_2^2 - v_1^2)$$

$$= \tfrac{1}{2} \times 1.056(160,000 - 10,000)$$

$$= 79,200 \text{ dyn/cm}^2$$

$$\approx 60 \text{ mmHg}$$

*Daniel Bernoulli, 1700–1782, a second-generation member of a Swiss family of 12 eminent mathematicians

Energy loss for arterial blood flow

- These ideal fluid circumstances for Bernoulli's equation do not apply to real fluid flow in the human circulation.
- This is due to energy loss from conversion of KE to heat, with a fall in pressure.

Laminar flow (Fig. 1.3a)

- In an ideal fluid, all layers move at the same velocity.
- The concept is that real fluids have an infinite number of layers, each sliding on the next, losing energy as they drag on each other.
- At low velocities, there are no cross-currents or eddy flow, with all layers moving in straight lines parallel to the vessel wall.
- The velocity of the layer of fluid immediately next to the vessel wall is zero. This is termed the 'no-slip condition'.
- Velocities of each layer away from the wall increase as resistance falls, with the peak velocity occurring in the layer at the center of the vessel.
- Blood viscosity increases as velocity decreases due to aggregation of red blood cells. Blood is therefore more viscous closer to the vessel wall than in the center of the vessel.
- Relatively stagnant flow may favor deposition of materials which leads to atherosclerosis or neointimal hyperplasia.

Plug flow (Fig. 1.3b)

- Flow with streamlined layers of fluid that have approximately the same velocity across the vessel lumen results in a blunt profile.
- It is usually seen with high-velocity flow such as with hemodynamically significant arterial stenosis.

a
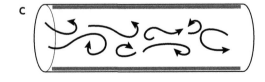

b
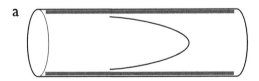

c
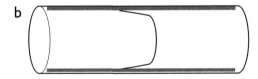

Fig. 1.3 *Flow profiles:*
a *Laminar flow.*
b *Plug flow.*
c *Turbulent flow.*

Viscosity, shear stress, and shear rate

- The coefficient of viscosity is determined by shear stress which reflects the force required to slide one layer on another, and shear rate which is dependent on flow:

$$\eta = T/D$$

$$T = 4\eta Q/\pi r^3$$

$$D = 4Q/\pi r^3$$

- In laminar flow, shear stress is least at the center of the vessel and strongest at the vessel wall.
- In straight segments of artery, flow is laminar and shear stress is directional and high.
- At relative arterial dilations, curvatures, angulations, branching or bifurcations, blood flow is disturbed with irregular distribution of low wall shear stress.
- Through the regulation of different processes of endothelial cells, high shear stress protects against atherosclerosis development whereas disturbed and low shear stress promote atherosclerosis deposition.
- Localized atherosclerotic deposition is most common at these sites of disturbed flow (see chapters about diseases of different regions of the body).

The boundary layer and boundary layer separation

- Boundary layers are layers of fluid in the immediate vicinity of the vessel wall where the effects of viscosity are significant.
- Boundary layers can be either laminar or turbulent with eddy currents.
- Reynolds' number is used to assess types of flow (see below).
- The boundary layer becomes thicker as the overall flow rate decreases or if the wall is rough causing disturbed flow, and relatively more KE is converted to heat.
- *Boundary layer separation* occurs when a portion of the boundary layer reverses in the direction of flow and this is disturbed flow.
- The 'separation point' is the point between forward and backward flow where shear stress is zero.
- Boundary layer separation can be seen when a vessel's diameter suddenly increases, resulting in a longer flow profile and a greater velocity gradient across the lumen.
- Boundary layer separation is well recognized from Doppler ultrasound in the internal carotid artery bulb (Fig. 1.4). It can also be observed at an arterial bypass graft anastomosis (Fig. 1.5) or just distal to a high-grade stenosis.
- Relative flow stasis in boundary layers and low shear forces trigger local atherosclerotic deposition.

Turbulence (Fig. 1.3c)

- Flow may become turbulent rather than streamlined when flow rate becomes great or when the flow passes through a stenosis or over a rough surface.
- Chaotic fluid movements in the form of eddy currents cause crosswise flow as well as flow along the vessel. This results in considerable energy loss and a fall in pressure that is not regained.
- This is maximal at each end of a stenosis.

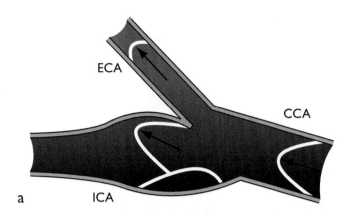

a

ICA

ECA

CCA

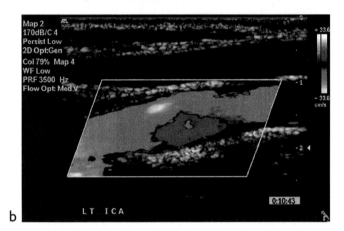

b

Fig. 1.4 *Boundary layer separation:*
a Boundary layer separation within the carotid bulb.
b Color Doppler image demonstrating boundary layer separation in the ICA bulb in a normal young patient. CCA, common carotid artery; ECA, external carotid artery; ICA, internal carotid artery.

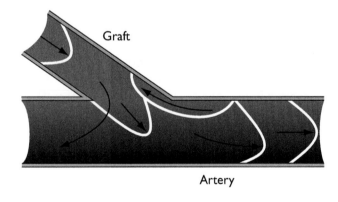

Graft

Artery

Fig. 1.5 *Boundary layer separation at an anastomosis site for a bypass graft.*

- The point at which flow breaks up is defined by *Reynolds' number.**

$$Re = vd\rho/\eta$$

- Re is more likely to be exceeded in large arteries and at high velocities.
- Turbulent flow can also occur when there is a localized decrease in diameter, such as with stenosis, causing an increase in velocity and a subsequent localized pressure fall.
- Flow is commonly turbulent for Re >2000.

*Osborne Reynolds, 1842–1912, British engineer and physicist

- This is more likely after exercise or vasodilator stimuli which reduce peripheral resistance.
- Laminar flow is silent whereas turbulent flow causes an audible bruit (see Chapter 3, page 31) or palpable thrill as with an arteriovenous fistula (see Chapter 13). These phenomena are due to the conversion of KE into sound or vibration energy.
- Turbulence causing a bruit may occur only with reduced peripheral resistance and increased velocity resulting from exercise.

Pulsatility due to cardiac activity

- Arterial flow signals combine forward flow from left ventricular contraction and reverse flow from tidal reflection (Fig. 1.6).
- The profile for flow changes throughout the pulse cycle is shown in Fig. 1.7.

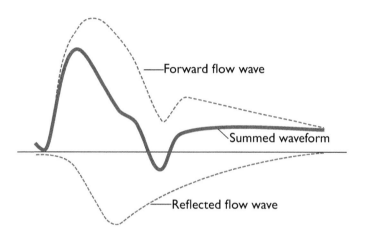

Forward flow wave

Summed waveform

Reflected flow wave

Fig. 1.6 *Arterial pulse.*
- *Upper curve – left ventricular contraction causes forward flow with a systolic and diastolic component.*
- *Lower curve – a water-hammer effect from flow striking major arterial branches as well as the peripheral resistance causes reverse flow.*
- *Middle curve – the actual flow signal is a summation of the two.*

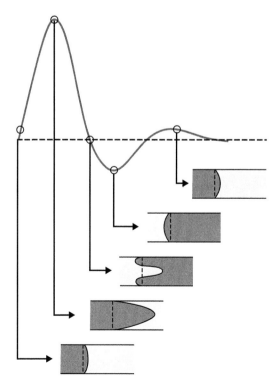

Fig. 1.7 *Flow profile.*
- *The profile is flat at the start of the pulse when flow is minimal, becomes parabolic through systole and then becomes mixed during diastole.*

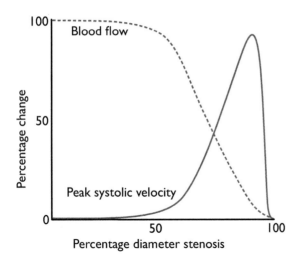

Fig. 1.8 *Flow and velocity changes related to severity of arterial stenosis.*

Pressure changes at an arterial stenosis (Fig. 1.2)
- These factors that lead to KE loss and pressure drop at a stenosis depend on the change in velocity between two points (1 and 2):

$$\Delta P = k(v_2 - v_1)^2$$

- Blood flow through an arterial stenosis starts to fall and the PSV rises when the diameter decreases to approximately 50%; there is a sharp late fall in the PSV to '*trickle flow*' beyond approximately 90–95% stenosis (Fig. 1.8).
- Flow becomes laminar again just beyond a stenosis but energy loss and fall in pressure persist.
- The value of the constant (k) depends more on shape than on length of stenosis and flow disturbance is greater if a stenosis is irregular.

Measuring an arterial percentage stenosis
- Stenosis can be defined by either reduced diameter or cross-sectional area:

$$\text{Diameter stenosis} = (1 - r_2/r_1) \times 100\%$$

$$\text{Cross-sectional area stenosis} = (1 - r_2^2/r_1^2) \times 100\%$$

- If the diameter is reduced by 50% then the area is reduced by 75%.

Resistance
- Resistance is determined by three factors:
  - ○ Viscosity of the fluid,
  - ○ Length of the vessel,
  - ○ Radius of the vessel.
- Resistance can be calculated by *Poiseuille's equation:**

$$R = 8\eta l/\pi r^4$$

- Radius is the most influential on resistance.
- Peripheral resistance is mostly controlled by the constriction and dilation of arterioles, and this in turn controls blood pressure.

---

*Jean-Louis-Marie Poiseuille, 1799–1869, French physician and physiologist

● Blood flow is inversely proportional to resistance.
● Resistance can also be calculated by *Ohm's law*:

$$R = \Delta P/Q$$

Resistance in parallel
● In parallel, resistance in each branch is greater than the resistance in the main pathway:

$$1/R_{TOTAL} = 1/R_1 + 1/R_2 + 1/R_3 + \dots$$

and

$$R_{TOTAL} = R'/N$$

Peripheral resistance
● Net resistance is less than the resistance of any single branch.
● The effect of branching on the net resistance depends on the following:
  ○ The radii of the branches – the smaller the radii of the branches compared with the main pathway, the greater the net resistance.
  ○ The number of branches – the smaller the number of branches, the greater the net resistance.
● Resistance is much higher in parallel smaller vessels so that the pressure drop occurs in the microcirculation rather than in larger arteries.
● Spectral Doppler shows the resistance in an arterial bed (Fig. 1.9).
● Blood flow to different organ beds is considered to be in parallel.
● Some sites such as the limbs and small intestine have an inherently *high resistance* and pulse reflection results in pulsatile flow with low, absent or reversed flow in diastole (Fig. 1.9a).
● Other organs such as the brain or kidneys have an inherently *low resistance*, resulting in relatively constant flow with forward flow throughout diastole (Fig. 1.9b).
● Stimuli for vasodilation of the arterioles cause resistance to fall in high-resistance circulations. Stimuli include normal activity such as exercise in limb muscles, sympathetic blockade in skin or food ingestion in the small intestine, and abnormal conditions include reactive hyperemia, inflammation, surgically created arteriovenous fistulas and tumors.
● In many regions, resistance vessels in the microcirculation constrict if pressure rises and dilate if pressure falls to maintain a relatively constant flow termed 'autoregulation'.

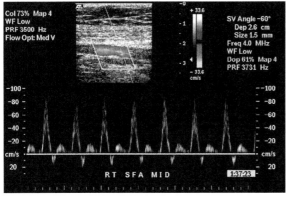
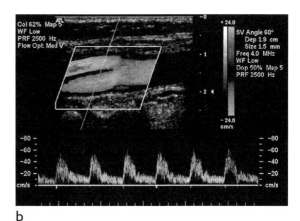

a   b

Fig. 1.9 *Spectral traces from an artery:*
a *High-resistance circulation.*
b *Low-resistance circulation.*

Collateral resistance

- Multiple parallel collaterals that develop around an occluded artery have a total resistance that is far higher than resistance in the normal native artery.
- However, collateral resistance around an arterial occlusion is less than peripheral resistance at rest, even allowing for pulses to be felt.
- Collateral resistance becomes greater than peripheral resistance if the latter is reduced by exercise, and the hyperemic response is then far less than in a normal circulation.
- Spectral waveforms proximal to high-grade stenoses or occlusions are high-resistance signals, whereas waveforms distal to these lesions are 'dampened' and low resistance (Fig. 1.10).

Blood flow through an arterial bypass graft

- The relative sizes of graft and collateral bed determine how well a graft functions. At rest, resistance from either is so much less than the peripheral resistance that almost any graft will carry adequate flow.
- It requires severe graft stenosis to cause a fall in pressure and flow.

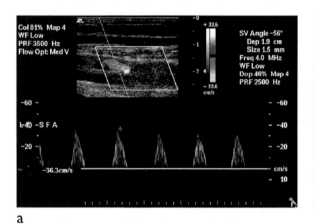 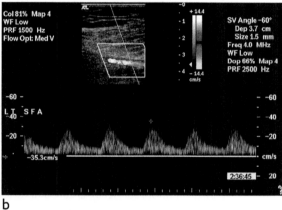

a b

Fig. 1.10 *Spectral traces in association with severe stenosis or occlusion:*
a *Proximal high-resistance signal.*
b *Distal dampened low-resistance signal.*

Resistances in series

- In series, resistance through each consecutive site is less than for the main channel alone:

$$R_{TOTAL} = R_1 + R_2 + R_3 + \ldots$$

- Resistance for each arterial stenosis combines to cause increased net resistance to flow.
- Multiple short stenoses cause a greater fall in perfusion pressure and velocity than one long stenosis alone.
- TPR is the combined resistance of the arteries, arterioles, capillaries, venules and veins.

Intermittent claudication

- At rest, circulation to muscles is a high-resistance system.
- During exercise, muscle contraction releases vasodilator chemicals which cause arteriolar dilation and blood flow increases some 10–20 times.

- After stopping exertion, potential pain-producing metabolites are washed away and vasodilation recedes within 30–60 seconds.
- An arterial occlusion or severe stenosis impedes the propagating pulse so that the peak increase in flow is much reduced (Fig. 1.11).
- Pain-producing metabolites accumulate above a threshold, causing pain referred to as intermittent claudication (*claudicare* – to limp).

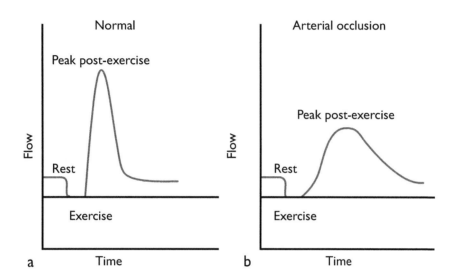

Fig. 1.11 *Blood flow in the calf after a period of exercise:*
a *Normal circulation.*
b *Limb with arterial occlusion or severe stenosis.*

Critical ischemia
- Unlike muscle, the skin circulation has very considerable sympathetic nervous control.
- Decreased perfusion pressure due to an arterial occlusion or severe stenosis is compensated by arteriolar dilation until disease is advanced.
- *Rest pain* – there comes a stage where skin circulation is reduced beyond a point where compensation can occur, and metabolites accumulate that cause severe burning pain in the foot. This first becomes apparent at night due to decreased perfusion from the normal nocturnal fall in systemic blood pressure.

Changes in the wall of an aneurysm
- Weakening in the wall allows it to progressively stretch and increase in diameter and length.
- Circumferential wall tension (Tc) in a cylindrical tube is defined by *LaPlace's law:**

$$Tc = \Delta Pr/t$$

- Wall tension increases as the radius increases and wall thickness decreases so as to allow more rapid expansion and eventual rupture.

*Pierre Simon LaPlace, 1749–1827, French mathematician and astronomer

BLOOD FLOW IN VEINS

Blood flow in lower limb veins
- Deep and superficial veins are connected by perforating veins at various levels.
- Reverse flow from gravity, inspiration or straining is normally prevented by venous valves, so that flow is only towards the heart.
- Valves become more numerous the further the vein is from the central circulation and are not present in the inferior vena cava or iliac veins.
- Perforators normally have valves that direct flow from superficial to deep veins.
- Deep veins carry more than 80% of the normal venous circulation.
- Venous blood pressure is steady and changes little during the cardiac cycle.
- Pulsatile contractions of the right atrium cause transient increase in venous pressure and arrest of flow which is restored as the atrium relaxes. This is observed only in central veins.
- There is phasic variation of flow with respiration in proximal veins in the limbs, although this is lost in distal veins.

Factors aiding venous return
- Veins offer little resistance to flow by having large-diameter lumina and being thin walled, but venous pressure alone is too low to provide adequate blood return, and there is only a small pressure gradient in the venous system to aid flow.
- Venous return is aided by the following:
  - The respiratory 'pump' – intra-abdominal and intrathoracic pressure changes during respiration compress veins
  - The muscular 'pump' – contraction of skeletal muscles compresses veins.
- Changing intrathoracic pressures due to respiration causes opposite effects in the upper and the lower limbs.
- For veins in the upper extremities, inspiration results in an increase in pressure gradient to central veins and venous flow increases.
- For veins in the lower extremities, inspiration causes the diaphragm to descend, increasing intra-abdominal pressure and causing venous flow to slow, whereas lower limb venous flow increases during expiration.
- Increased intra-abdominal and intrathoracic pressure with straining or the Valsalva maneuver causes flow to slow or stop in all limbs.

Venous blood flow velocity and resistance
- Venous flow is increased by vasodilation with exercise and reduced by vasoconstriction caused by cold or arterial insufficiency.
- Most resistance in veins is due to surrounding tissues and the above-described changes in intrathoracic and intra-abdominal pressures.
- Just as for branching arteries, resistance in smaller veins in parallel is greater than resistance in a large vein such as the inferior vena cava.
- Accordingly, the larger the vein, the greater the flow velocity.
- Blood flow is most stagnant in smaller veins such as in the calf making them more susceptible to venous thrombosis.

2 VASCULAR PATHOLOGY

Occlusive arterial disease is most commonly due to atherosclerosis. Aneurysmal arterial disease may have a different pathogenesis. There are several uncommon or rare non-atherosclerotic arterial diseases. Venous thrombosis and chronic venous disease are also discussed.

NORMAL ARTERIAL STRUCTURE AND FUNCTION
- The wall of a large artery has three layers (Fig. 2.1).
- Ultrasound can distinguish the three layers (Fig. 2.2a) and measure intima–media thickness (IMT), which relates well to future risk for clinical arterial disease.

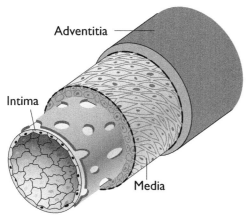

Fig. 2.1 *Three layers of an arterial wall.*
Adapted from Fig. 12.2a, Myers KA, Marshall RD, Freidin J. Principles of Pathology. Oxford: Blackwell, 1980. Reproduced with permission from Blackwell.

Intima
- It is a single layer of endothelial cells.
- It is supported by a basement membrane and internal elastic lamina.
- These cells regulate blood clotting and vascular tone.

Media
- It contains smooth muscle cells (SMCs).
- These maintain vascular tone and synthesize connective tissue.

Adventitia
- This consists of fibroblasts in a matrix of collagen and glycoproteins.

ATHEROSCLEROSIS
Etiology
- It involves blood contents, endothelial cells and SMCs in the media.
- Endothelial injury activates white blood cells, platelets and endothelial cells to cause biochemical changes in the underlying media.

- SMCs react by migrating from the media into the subendothelial plane.
- SMCs proliferate and change from contractile cells to cells synthesizing lipid-rich foam.
- Secondary degeneration releases lipid and platelets aggregate on the surface.

Risk factors
- There is an inherent risk for atherosclerosis to varying degrees in all humans.
- The severity and rate of progression are accentuated by several risk factors:
  - Smoking,
  - Diabetes mellitus,
  - Hypertension,
  - Hyperlipidemia,
  - Homocystinemia.

Pathology
- Lesions tend to be patchy and concentrated at common sites.
- Disease is more pronounced where flow is relatively stagnant against the arterial wall such as the aortic or carotid bifurcation.
- This allows more prolonged contact of injurious agents with the wall.
- Evolution of atheromatous lesions can be demonstrated by B-mode ultrasound (Fig. 2.2).

The fatty streak
- This early phase with subendothelial aggregation of lipid-rich foam cells occurs from childhood.

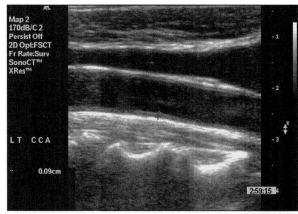

a

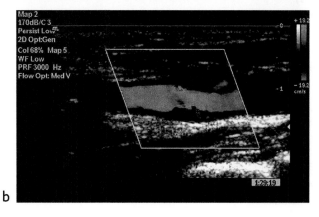

b

Fig. 2.2 Ultrasound appearances of normal arterial wall and atheromatous plaques.
a Layers of a normal arterial wall showing intima–media thickness, best measured on the far wall.
b A lipid-rich plaque resulting in a homogeneous echolucent appearance, apparent as a filling defect only with color Doppler.

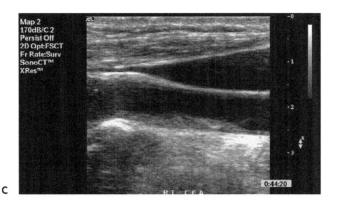

c

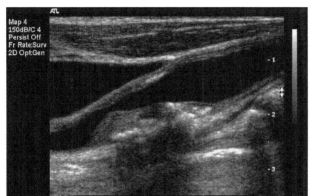

d

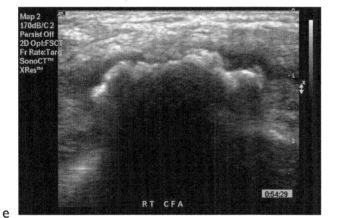

e

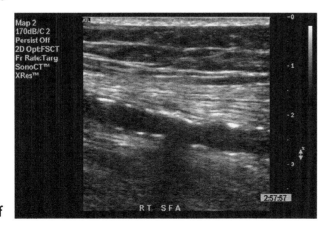

f

Fig. 2.2 (continued)
c *A diffusely fibrous plaque resulting in a homogeneous echogenic appearance.*
d *A plaque containing various combinations of lipid, fibrous tissue, and calcification resulting in a heterogeneous plaque.*
e *'Cauliflower' calcification causing acoustic shadowing.*
f *Diffuse calcification causing plaques along a considerable length of artery.*

Fibrous plaques
- These more advanced lesions have aggregates of subendothelial SMCs surrounded by connective tissue and lipid.
- They are covered by a fibrous cap.

Atheromas
- The next stage contains lipid that accumulates as foam cells break down.
- Vasa vasora in the base of the plaque may hemorrhage into its core, increasing its size.
- The swollen plaque may rupture, discharging its contents into the lumen and leaving a surface ulcer.
- Plaque content and platelet aggregates form a potential source of emboli.

Calcified plaques
- Secondary degeneration can then cause an inflammatory response, with repair leading to a mixed lesion of fibrous tissue, lipid and secondary calcification.
- The irregular surface may cause thrombus and platelets to aggregate and embolize.
- However, there is less lipid and a reduced risk of plaque rupture.

Arterial thrombosis
- The final stage may be precipitated by plaque rupture to release contents that promote occlusion by thrombosis.
- Alternately, progressive degeneration can cause the arterial lumen to narrow and eventually occlude.
- Unlike veins, there is no inherent mechanism for spontaneous thrombolysis.
- Recanalization of occluded arteries is rare.

Pathological sequela
- Acute thrombosis can result from minor to moderate stenosis to cause acute ischemia as the first presentation.
- Disease must narrow an artery to a 'critical stenosis' before significant symptoms develop.
- Critical stenosis or chronic occlusion leads to chronic ischemia.
- Occlusion extends between major branches that connect to form collateral arteries around the occlusion.
- The severity of symptoms in part depends on how well collaterals form.
- Particles from atheromas or secondary surface thrombus can detach to cause patchy infarcts from embolism.

ARTERIAL ANEURYSMS

Etiology
- Degenerative aneurysms can affect any major artery.
- There are several predisposing factors:
  - Deficiencies of enzymes responsible for collagen cross-linking.
  - Impaired oxygen diffusion to the arterial wall through an intraluminal thrombus to cause hypoxic necrosis.
  - Familial history: family clusters occur and first-degree male relatives are four times more likely to develop an aneurysm.

- There are other types of aneurysms:
  - Aneurysms associated with inflammatory arteritis.
  - Mycotic aneurysms from infection in the artery wall.
  - Traumatic aneurysms.

Risk factors

- Family history.
- Hypertension.
- Smoking.
- Chronic obstructive pulmonary disease.
- Atherosclerotic arterial disease elsewhere.
- Unlike atherosclerosis, diabetes is not a risk factor.

Pathology (Fig. 2.3)

Fusiform and saccular aneurysms

- Collagen and elastin in the wall degenerate and calcium is deposited. Atherosclerotic lesions make the remaining wall weak and brittle.
- Tangential stress from intravascular pressure is greater at certain sites predisposing to local dilation.
- Laminated thrombus accumulates on the degenerated inner arterial wall.
- Elastic retraction is lost, the diameter progressively increases and the aneurysmal artery also becomes more elongated and tortuous.

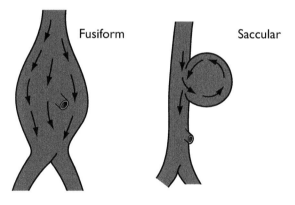

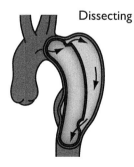

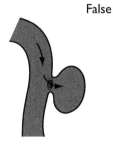

Fig. 2.3 *Types of aneurysms:*
- *Fusiform involving the entire circumference of the aortic wall.*
- *Saccular involving just a portion of the aortic circumference.*
- *Dissecting with a false lumen.*
- *False aneurysm from arterial trauma.*

From Fig. 13.10, Queral L. In: Bergan JJ, Yao JS. Surgery of the Aorta and its Body Branches. New York: Grune & Stratton, 1979. Reproduced with permission.

Dissecting aneurysm

- Aortic dissection can commence with a tear in the intima from the start of the aortic arch, from just beyond the left subclavian artery or less frequently from within the abdominal aorta or internal carotid artery.
- It is due to necrosis in the media and is common in diseases with congenital collagen deficiency – Marfan's* or Ehlers–Danlos** syndrome.
- Presentation may be acute with occlusion of aortic branches or iliac arteries, or chronic with aneurysm formation.

False aneurysm

- Accidental or iatrogenic arterial trauma can cause a defect in the artery wall.
- Hemorrhage leads to a local hematoma.
- Arterial pressure can keep the opening patent to progressively form an aneurysmal space, compressing the hematoma against adjacent tissues.

NON-ATHEROSCLEROTIC ARTERIAL DISEASES

- Several uncommon non-atherosclerotic arterial diseases should be considered, particularly in younger patients who lack major risk factors for atherosclerosis.

Inflammatory arterial diseases

- Several diseases, probably caused by an immune reaction, have similar pathology but different clinical presentations.
- They may be distinguished by ultrasound, but most require arteriography or arterial biopsy for diagnosis.

Takayasu's ('pulseless') disease***

- This is common in Asia and affects children and young adults with a marked female preponderance.
- Inflammation affects all layers of the thoracic and abdominal aorta and its major branches.
- An acute inflammatory phase with nonspecific 'rheumatic-like' illness is followed years later by a chronic fibrotic phase which leads to large artery stenoses or occlusion, and aneurysms in some 30%.

Buerger's disease (thromboangiitis obliterans)****

- The disease usually occurs in young males, particularly from southern and eastern Europe, Israel, or Asia and always in smokers.
- An early acute phase shows inflammation in the arterial and venous walls and surrounding tissues causing thrombotic occlusion.
- This is followed by a chronic phase with fibrosis and collateral formation.
- Approximately 60% have lower limb symptoms, 30% have upper limb symptoms and 10% have both.
- However, arteriography shows changes in most arteries of all limbs indicating that disease is more extensive than predicted from symptoms.

---

*Antoine Bernard-Jean Marfan, 1858–1942, French pediatrician ***Mikito Takayasu, 1860–1938, Japanese ophthalmologist

**Edvard Lauritis Ehlers, 1863–1937, Danish dermatologist ****Leo Buerger, 1879–1943, Austrian-American surgeon

**Henri-Alexandre Danlos, 1844–1912, French dermatologist

Temporal (giant cell) arteritis

- This predominantly affects females, is found in most countries and is almost exclusively confined to the white population.
- The disease particularly affects temporal arteries but can occur in arteries to the extremities.

Behçet's disease*

- The condition is most prevalent in young males from eastern Mediterranean countries or Japan.
- The pathology is nonspecific inflammation in small and large vessels.
- Major arterial or venous thrombosis can occur at any site.
- Aneurysms particularly affect large arteries or sites of surgical anastomosis or arterial puncture.
- Disease is frequently at multiple sites.

Scleroderma

- There is adventitial fibrosis that usually affects small arteries in the hands, leading to Raynaud's phenomenon (see Chapter 5).
- It can also cause occlusion of large arteries to the limbs as a result of intimal hyperplasia.

Intrinsic diseases of the arterial wall
Aortic coarctation

- This is a congenital segment of aortic hypoplasia, often with associated visceral and renal artery stenosis.
- It can involve the thoracic or occasionally the proximal abdominal aorta.
- It occurs in young patients presenting with hypertension, impaired renal function, an aortic bruit and lower limb ischemia.

Fibromuscular dysplasia

- This usually involves one or both renal arteries (see Chapter 7), but can affect other visceral arteries, extracranial internal carotid arteries or external iliac arteries.
- Most patients are female aged <60 years.
- There is a series of stenoses with intervening dilations.

Arterial trauma
Acute arterial trauma

- Penetration through the arterial wall leads to major hemorrhage.
- However, many injuries rupture the intima and media leaving the adventitia intact.
- This can cause arterial occlusion and ischemia.
- In very large arteries, the lumen may remain patent and the weakened wall becomes aneurysmal.

Repetitive arterial trauma

- This can cause subintimal fibrosis with stenosis, degeneration with aneurysm formation or thrombotic occlusion.

---

*Hulusi Behçet, 1889–1948, Turkish dermatologist

Iatrogenic trauma
- Arterial catheterization for arteriography.
- Intra-arterial infusions of therapeutic agents.
- Thrombosed arterial reconstructions.

Post-irradiation arteritis
- Irradiation can cause endothelial damage in major arteries, usually manifest more than 1–2 years after treatment.
- Consequent fibrosis extends through the wall, causing arterial stenosis or occlusion.

Ergotism
- Oral or intravenous ergot administration can cause spasm of large arteries to the limbs or aortic arch branches.
- Spasm in the early stages is completely reversible within a few hours of stopping the drug but endothelial damage can lead to thrombosis.

VENOUS THROMBOSIS

Virchow's triad* (Fig. 2.4)
- Venous thrombosis results from combinations of three processes:
  - Stasis of blood flow,
  - Endothelial injury,
  - Activation of clotting.

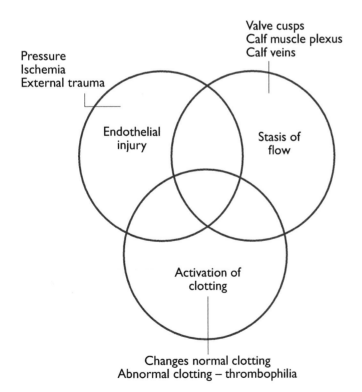

Fig. 2.4 *Virchow's triad.*

---

*Rudolf Ludwig Karl Virchow, 1821–1902, German pathologist

Venous thrombosis from hematological abnormalities

- *Hyperviscosity* due to hematological diseases that increase levels of red cells, white cells or serum proteins such as polycythemia, lymphomas or leukemias, or globulin disorders
- *Thrombophilia* associated with clotting factor abnormalities:
  - Deficiencies of normal clotting factors such as antithrombin III, protein C, or protein S.
  - Presence of abnormal clotting factors such as factor V Leiden, prothrombin gene mutation, antiphospholipid antibodies, or homocysteine.

Manifestations of venous thromboembolism

- Superficial thrombophlebitis (STP).
- Deep vein thrombosis (DVT), particularly in the lower limbs.
- Pulmonary embolism (PE).

Risk factors

Surgery

- Common cause, particularly after lower limb orthopedic operations
- Factors during surgery that increase risk include poor hydration, immobility, a prolonged operation and deep anesthesia.

Intravenous lines and catheters

- Devices used to infuse nutrients or drugs are often required for long periods and are subject to a risk of causing thrombosis.
- This is a particular problem in the upper limbs.

Pregnancy

- DVT occurs in fewer than 1 in 1,000 pregnancies but PE is a leading cause of maternal mortality.
- DVT is more common after a cesarean section and with advanced maternal age or obesity.

Oral contraceptives and hormone replacement therapy

- Both low-dose estrogen oral contraceptives and progestogens for hormone replacement therapy increase the risk, particularly during the first year.

Medical diseases

- Myocardial infarction, heart failure, stroke, respiratory disease or cancer leads to a high risk of DVT, increased by age or chemotherapy.

Thrombophilia

- Approximately 25% of patients with idiopathic DVT have thrombophilia.
- Thrombosis due to thrombophilia often occurs only under other high-risk conditions.

Extended travel

- Thrombosis due to stasis associated with inactivity during long-haul travel.
- Approximately two-thirds have associated medical disorders, hormone prescription or thrombophilia.

SUPERFICIAL VENOUS DISEASE

- It is necessary to understand normal lower limb venous circulation (Fig. 2.5) to be able to understand the hemodynamic changes in superficial venous disease (Fig. 2.6).
- It manifests as varicose veins which can lead to complications.
- There is debate about whether this is a descending or an ascending process.
- The descending hypothesis is that the hydrostatic pressure distends previously normal veins.
- The ascending hypothesis is that primary degeneration in the vein wall, starting in distal branches, allows normal pressures to dilate these abnormal veins.
- Either way, valves at junctions between deep and superficial veins become incompetent allowing reflux to occur down the superficial veins and into varicose tributaries.
- This then becomes a progressive process.
- A primary cause for degenerative changes in the vein walls is unknown.
- Risk factors that lead to progression include obesity, multiparity and prolonged standing.

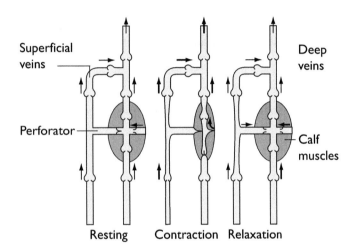

Fig. 2.5 *Flow with muscle contraction in the normal venous circulation.*
- *Resting – blood flows so that valves are open and pressure in the vein is the hydrostatic pressure from the heart.*
- *Contraction – blood is expelled from deep veins towards the heart.*
- *Relaxation – valves close and blood cannot reflux into deep or superficial veins, pressure in deep veins falls, pressure is higher in superficial veins, and blood flows from superficial to deep veins through the saphenous junctions and perforators.*
- *Blood enters through the microcirculation but usually with insufficient time to refill deep veins before the next muscle contraction, so that ambulatory venous pressure remains well below the hydrostatic pressure.*

Adapted from Fig. 129-17, Sumner DS. In: Rutherford RB. Vascular Surgery. Philadelphia: WB Saunders, 1995. Reproduced with permission.

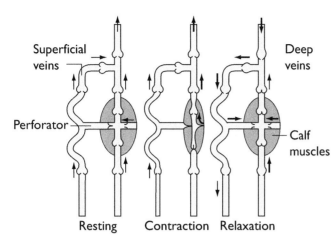

Fig. 2.6 *Flow with muscle contraction in limbs that have superficial venous reflux and varicose veins.*
- *Resting – blood flows so that valves are open and pressure in a vein is the hydrostatic pressure from the heart.*
- *Contraction – blood is expelled from deep veins towards the heart and out to the surface through incompetent perforators.*
- *Relaxation – blood flows retrogradely through incompetent connections into superficial veins and varices, and a pressure gradient causes blood to flow inwards through perforators from distended superficial veins to emptied deep veins.*
- *Deep veins fill at a greater rate and ambulatory venous pressure in deep and superficial veins is higher than normal.*

Adapted from Fig. 129-12, Sumner DS. In: Rutherford RB. Vascular Surgery. Philadelphia: WB Saunders, 1995. Reproduced with permission.

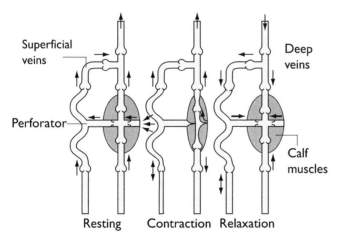

Fig. 2.7 *Flow with muscle contraction in limbs with deep venous reflux.*
- *Resting – blood flows so that valves are open and pressure in the veins is the hydrostatic pressure from the heart.*
- *Contraction – blood is expelled from deep veins towards the heart and out through perforators to the superficial veins under high pressure.*
- *Relaxation – blood immediately flows backwards past incompetent valves; there is no pressure gradient between distended superficial veins and deep veins, and blood pools in both.*
- *Deep veins fill immediately and ambulatory venous pressure in deep and superficial veins is equal to the hydrostatic pressure.*

Adapted from Fig. 129-20, Sumner DS. In: Rutherford RB. Vascular Surgery. Philadelphia: WB Saunders, 1995. Reproduced with permission.

DEEP VENOUS REFLUX (FIG. 2.7)

- Valves in deep veins may be congenitally absent, present but not functioning, or destroyed by past DVT with recanalization.
- This leads to more severe venous hypertension, and risk of damage to the skin and fat distally referred to as lipodermatosclerosis.

DEEP VENOUS OBSTRUCTION

- Thrombus in a deep vein may fail to recanalize, leading to long-term chronic obstruction.
- Pressures in deep veins increase with calf muscle contraction, forcing blood to pass out through perforators, leading to severe superficial venous hypertension.
- Saphenous veins and their major tributaries are collaterals for outflow and cannot be removed for fear of further restricting outflow and worsening symptoms.

PERFORATORS

- A frequent observation while scanning is detection of dilated perforating veins that join superficial and deep veins.
- Normally, these have valves that direct flow from superficial to deep.
- When dilated, valve function is lost and blood can flow in either direction.
- There is debate about whether or not outward flow in these perforators contributes to superficial venous hypertension.
- It is generally agreed that blood can be ejected through perforators under high pressure with calf muscle contraction if there is deep venous reflux with pooling in the deep veins.
- However, many phlebologists contend that it is likely that this does not contribute to superficial venous hypertension if there is no deep venous reflux and pooling.
- In this situation, it is more likely that the perforators are dilated as a result of high flow from superficial varices into deep veins.
- This view is supported by the frequent observation that the dilated perforators return to normal after treatment to eliminate superficial varices.

3 PERFORMING A SCAN

Vascular ultrasound combines various modalities to study blood vessels and blood flow (Fig. 3.1). Continuous-wave Doppler is the simplest technique for evaluation. Ultrasound machines use pulsed-wave ultrasound combining B-mode and pulsed Doppler as the duplex scanner. This chapter assumes that the reader has a full grasp of ultrasound physics principles which are explained in depth in relevant dedicated textbooks.

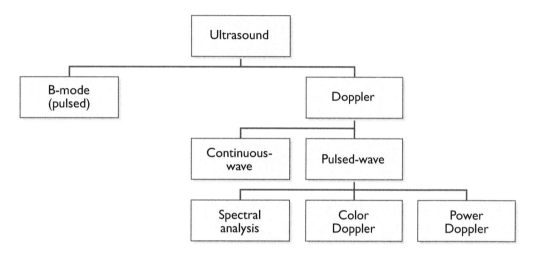

Fig. 3.1 *Modalities used in vascular ultrasound to study blood vessels and blood flow.*

CONTROLS FOR ULTRASOUND MACHINES

- Ultrasound machines have a preset menu for each anatomical site although some sonographers prefer to create their own settings.
- Machines made by different manufacturers may have different names for the controls but they all serve the same purpose.
- Some machines do not have all of the functions listed whereas others have controls not mentioned here.

Monitor controls and displays
- Brightness
- Contrast
- Color velocity scale
- Patient annotation
- Mechanical and thermal indices
- Time gain compensation (TGC) curve
- Focal zones
- Depth scale

- Transducer frequency
- Color and B-mode parameters.

Keyboard functions
- Annotations
- Transducer select key
- Setup select keys
- Function select keys
- Output/power
- Frame-capture capabilities and cine-loop
- Calculations – distances between objects, velocities, and various ratios.

B-mode controls
- TGC/depth gain compensation (DGC)/time sensitivity control (TSC)
- Sector width
- Singular and multiple focal zones
- Depth of field of view
- Gain
- Pre- and post-processing zoom
- Dynamic range (compression curves)
- Gray-scale maps
- B-mode chroma
- Pulse repetition frequency (PRF)
- Persistence/frame averaging/smoothing.

Color Doppler controls
- Baseline
- Color write priority
- Frequency range
- Color box position, size, and angle
- Color maps
- Wall filter
- Gain
- Color invert
- Persistence/frame averaging/smoothing.

Spectral Doppler controls
- Baseline
- Spectral invert
- Gain
- Sample volume size, position, and angle
- Wall filter
- Sweep speed
- Doppler chroma.

Power Doppler controls

- Baseline
- Power write priority
- Power box size, position, and angle
- Power Doppler maps
- Wall filter
- Persistence.

BASIC PRINCIPLES OF SOME ULTRASOUND VARIABLES

- *PRF* – the frequency for emitting pulses from the transducer (kHz).
- *TGC* – echoes from different depths can be suppressed or enhanced, particularly enhancement for otherwise attenuated deeper signals, to provide even brightness throughout the depth of view.
- *Dynamic range* – the range of echo brightness levels displayed. If the dynamic range is reduced (compression increased), lower-level echoes are suppressed allowing greater contrast of higher-intensity signals. This is a pre-processing function so that if low-level echoes are to be examined, the area must be re-imaged with a higher dynamic range.
- *Compression curves* – these manipulate the way in which echo brightness is stored and assigned shades of gray on the display. This is a post-processing function so that the image does not have to be rescanned.
- *Line density* – number of lines composing the image.
- *Field of view* – the depth and width of the image displayed on the screen.
- *Frame rate* – each frame is erased when the process has completed a field of view and the screen is refreshed with a new image. This frame rate is set to produce what appears to be continuous real-time scanning. The display can be frozen at any time.
- *Frame averaging/persistence* – averages the brightness or color allocated to each pixel over more than one frame. Increased persistence smoothes the appearance of real-time images. The apparent frame rate is slowed even though the actual frame rate remains unchanged.
- *Echo/write priority* – when color or power Doppler is activated, the control is set at a level that determines whether echoes with brightness greater than the threshold are displayed only in B-mode whereas echoes with brightness less than the threshold are color coded.
- *Focal zone* – a focused ultrasound beam is narrower than an unfocused beam would be from a comparable transducer. The reduction in beam width occurs only within the focal zone.
- *Zoom* – magnifies a region of interest in the image. Read zoom is purely a magnification process; the zoomed region still uses the same number of pixels per area of patient as the unzoomed image. It is a post-processing function. Write zoom is a pre-processing function that increases the number of pixels per area of patient.

B-MODE ECHOGENICITY

- This is the gray-scale level assigned to each pixel and represents the acoustic impedance mismatch at interfaces.
- Gray-scale echoes range from bright to dark according to the amount of reflection.
- A structure that returns echoes is *echoic* and if no echoes are returned then the area is *anechoic*.
- A strong reflector is represented as being bright and is *hyperechoic*, and a weak reflector is shown as being dark or *hypoechoic*.
- An area in the image that shows reflections is referred to as *echogenic* and an area that shows absent reflections is *echolucent*.
- A structure that has a relatively uniform echogenicity is referred to as *homogeneous*, whether it be echogenic or hypoechoic.
- A structure with variable echogenicity is referred to as *heterogeneous*, containing both echogenic and echolucent areas or echoes of varying brightness.

Tissue characteristics that affect echogenicity
- Reflection and scattering at acoustic interfaces.
- Attenuation and absorption.
- Depth of the reflector.

Technical considerations that determine echogenicity
- Gain.
- Transducer frequency.
- TGC.
- Dynamic range.

DETECTING ARTERIAL STENOSIS

Aliasing
- Aliasing or Doppler shift ambiguity can occur with pulsed Doppler if there is a high velocity at an arterial stenosis.
- It occurs if the Doppler shift exceeds the Nyquist* limit.
- With spectral Doppler, high frequencies are 'wrapped around' and appear to be in the opposite direction relative to the baseline (Fig. 3.2).
- With color Doppler, aliasing affects each pixel in the color box where velocities are higher than the Nyquist limit, and this produces regions of reversed color (Fig. 3.3) which can be confused with true reverse flow or turbulence.
- From the Doppler equation:

$$f_{max} = 2f_o v_{max} \cos\theta / c = PRF/2$$

so that:

$$v_{max} = cPRF/4f_o \cos\theta$$

---

*Harry Nyquist, 1889–1976, Swedish Scientist

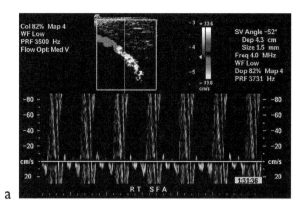

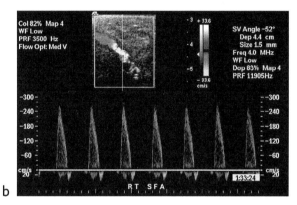

Fig. 3.2 *Aliasing shown by spectral Doppler:*
a *Aliasing is easily recognized because the peak is shown in the opposite direction.*
b *Increasing the velocity scale eliminates aliasing to restore a complete signal.*

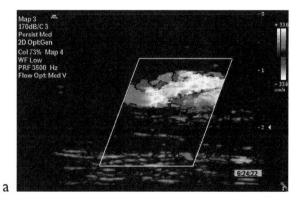

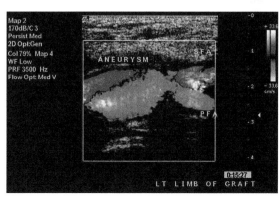

Fig. 3.3 *Aliasing shown by color Doppler:*
a *Aliasing shows pale-red and pale-blue high-frequency colors without a dark line between because there is no phase of zero flow.*
b *True flow reversal shows a fine dark line of demarcation between deep red and blue low-frequency colors.*

- This shows that there are several ways to reduce aliasing with pulsed Doppler:
  - Increase the velocity scale (PRF)
  - Reduce the transmitted frequency f_o
  - Increase the angle of insonation θ (decrease $\cos\theta$)
  - Move the baseline.
  - Ultrasound machines can use an automated technique to avoid aliasing:
    - Echoes can be received from two sample volume depths, the deeper from the vessel of interest and the superficial not in a vessel.
    - The machine is programmed to sense that a pulse must be emitted and received before the next pulse is emitted.
    - A high PRF is used to make it appear that the reflected signal comes from the more superficial sample even though the Doppler shift comes from the deeper sample.

Spectral waveform flow characteristics

- Flow through a non-stenotic region is laminar (see Chapter 1, page 4) with a clean spectral window (Fig. 3.4a).
- Disturbed non-laminar flow causing spectral broadening will occur as velocity of flow increases through a stenosis (Fig. 3.4b).
- As the severity of stenosis increases, flow will become turbulent (see Chapter 1, page 5) (Fig. 3.4c).
- There will be dampened flow proximal and just distal to a high-grade stenosis and increased velocities with spectral broadening or turbulence within the stenotic jet. Within a few centimeters distal to the stenosis flow will be of low resistance (Fig. 3.5).

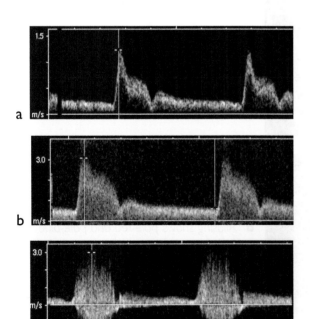

Fig. 3.4 *Spectral waveform characteristics:*
a *Laminar flow.*
b *Disturbed flow.*
c *Turbulent flow.*

Image kindly supplied by Martin Necas, Hamilton, New Zealand.

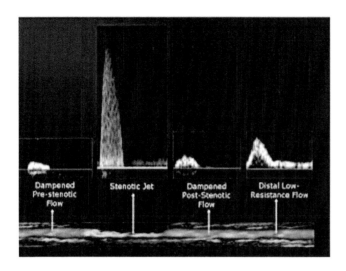

Fig. 3.5 *Spectral waveform characteristics in association with a high-grade stenosis.*

Image kindly supplied by Martin Necas, Hamilton, New Zealand.

Bruit

- Turbulent flow in an artery causes the vessel wall to vibrate and this produces a noise (bruit) to propagate through tissues that can be heard with a stethoscope or seen on an ultrasound scan as a color mosaic pattern (Fig. 3.6).

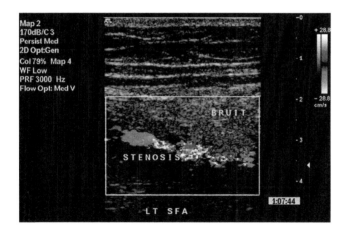

Fig. 3.6 *Bruit.*
- *Color signals in tissues due to reverberations from the arterial wall at a site of turbulence corresponding to an arterial bruit.*

HOW TO OPTIMIZE THE IMAGE

- It is usual practice to initially orient anatomy and view pathology using *B-mode*, to proceed to qualitatively examine blood flow and flow abnormalities with *color Doppler*, and to then quantitatively assess whether flow is normal or disturbed with *spectral Doppler*.
- Principles relating to all ultrasound studies are discussed in this section.
- Principles specific to various regions are discussed in the chapters covering the diseases of different areas of the body.

All modalities
- Select the appropriate transducer.
- Apply copious gel.
- Avoid excessive transducer pressure.
- Select windows where vessels are most superficial.
- Find windows through soft tissues with uniform density and low acoustic impedance such as muscle, avoiding fat and strong reflectors such as gas or bone.
- Move the patient into different positions or take advantage of a tilt table.
- Increase power as a last resort (ALARA – as low as reasonably achievable).

B-mode
- Position the focal zone just deep to the area of interest. This decreases beam thickness and therefore improves lateral resolution at the level of interest.
- If possible, insonate vessels at 90° for maximum specular reflection to give best definition of the vessel wall, atheromatous plaque or thrombus.
- To ensure correct gain, image a 'clear' section of the vessel lumen in longitudinal, increase gain until the lumen fills with noise and then decrease gain until the lumen becomes clear of noise and black in appearance.
- Adjust TGC throughout the duration of the scan.
- Reduce the scanning depth to increase the frame rate and decrease signal attenuation.

Color Doppler
- Increase the color gain and echo-write priority to a level where there is good color filling of vessels but no color bleeding.
- Reduce the width of the color box to increase the frame rate.
- Steer the color box or 'heel and toe' the transducer to avoid insonating the vessel of interest at 90° because otherwise Doppler shifts will not be coded.
- Change to a higher-frequency transducer to increase Doppler shifts if low-velocity flow is suspected but cannot be color-coded.

Spectral Doppler
- Set power and gain low and adjust levels up from the minimum until the optimum signal is achieved with the least surrounding background noise. This helps distinguish true spectral broadening from artifact.
- Initially, set the wall filter on minimum to ensure that low velocities are not omitted from the spectral trace.
- 'Heel and toe' the transducer to ensure that the Doppler angle is always ≤60°.
- Increase sample size when analyzing low velocities to allow more time for Doppler shifts to be detected.
- Use 'micromovements' to ensure that the sample volume remains in the center of the vessel.

TIPS!

- Standardize how images are displayed in transverse and longitudinal views (Fig. 3.7).
- If there is a stenosis with an eccentric jet stream, place the cursor parallel to the actual flow direction shown by color Doppler and not parallel to the vessel wall (see Fig. 6.24).
- Use the adjacent vein as a guide if the artery is occluded.

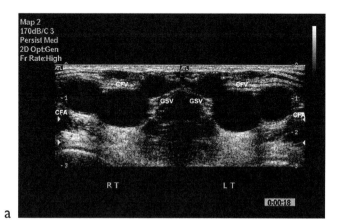

a

b

Fig. 3.7 *Image orientation – personal practice.*

- *There is usually an orientation marker on the transducer and a corresponding orientation icon on the image.*
- *If the icon is not present it is assumed to be on the left of the screen.*
- *Orient yourself by using known landmarks.*
- **a** Transverse view: *hold the transducer so that the patient's image is facing towards you. When scanning the saphenofemoral junction, the medial aspect will be on the right of the screen for the right lower limb and the left for the left lower limb.*
- **b** Longitudinal view: *hold the transducer so that the cephalad end is to the left of the screen. When scanning femoral arteries, the common femoral is to the left of the screen and the superficial femoral and profunda femoris arteries are to the right.*

LIMITATIONS

All studies

- It can be difficult to obtain the best angle for insonation and Doppler sampling.
- The color display is in two dimensions whereas flow is three dimensional.
- The short time required to rapidly and repetitively switch from B-mode to spectral Doppler reduces the frame rate for B-mode and PRF for pulsed Doppler.

- The small sample size for spectral Doppler provides information for only a small segment in the larger field of view.
- The sample volume for spectral Doppler is shown on a frozen B-mode image but the signal will be reduced or lost if the transducer or patient moves. The Doppler shift displayed is also affected if the transducer's 'heel-and-toe' angle is changed after the image is frozen. These can be overcome by using B-mode and spectral Doppler in real time.
- Displayed flow may be generated from different times within the cardiac cycle due to time delays required to produce a complete color image.
- Decreasing the range gate size improves axial resolution but decreases sensitivity due to reduced signal-to-noise ratio.
- Decreasing the beam thickness reduces the transit time for red blood cells to cross the beam so that sampling time is decreased, causing uncertainty for Doppler shift readings.
- Scarring from previous surgery can cause increased beam attenuation.
- A 90° insonation angle prevents color filling of vessels.
- Scanning can be difficult if the patient is elderly, large, incapacitated or unable to move.

Intra-abdominal studies
- Obesity can lead to loss of signal beyond a depth of 13–18 cm.
- Gas pockets in the stomach or bowel will produce acoustic shadows.
- Calcification and scar tissue from previous surgery can cause shadowing or extensive beam attenuation.
- It is difficult to compress abdominal veins. Use color Doppler to follow the veins because loss of color flow may suggest occlusive thrombus.
- Respiratory motion may make it difficult to capture a spectral Doppler signal. Be prepared to ask the patient to hold his or her breath.
- Vessels may be obscured by an abdominal aortic aneurysm.

Arterial studies
- Tortuous vessels can cause difficulties in obtaining Doppler angles <60°.
- Tortuosity can cause apparent velocity increase, although there is no stenosis present.
- For lower limb arterial studies, scanning can be difficult if the patient has had an amputation or recent surgery or has ulcers or gangrene.
- Calcification of vessels can cause extensive beam attenuation.

Extracranial cerebrovascular studies
- It can be difficult to communicate with a patient who has had a stroke causing deficits that affect speech, movement, memory or even consciousness.

Venous studies
- The age of thrombus can be difficult to define.
- Color Doppler can obscure partial thrombus if color gain and echo-write priority are set too high.
- Veins to be studied can be obscured by overlying ulceration.
- It can be difficult to compress veins at deep sites or if there is pain from thrombus.
- Low flow within a partially recanalized vein can be difficult to detect.

Vessels of the thoracic outlet

- There can be a rich collateral system making identification of vessels difficult.
- Interference by bony structures, both through poor transducer-to-skin contact and acoustic shadowing obscuring vessels.
- Subclavian vessels can have a mirror image deep to the high impedance mismatch of the pleura–lung interface.
- A normal nerve is easily mistaken for a chronically thrombosed brachial vein.
- Deep veins of the forearm are small and can be difficult to see.

REGIONAL ULTRASOUND STUDIES

- The following sections discuss general principles for studying intra-abdominal vessels, extracranial and lower limb arteries, lower limb veins and upper limb vessels.
- This includes preparing the patient for the study, selecting appropriate transducers, setting up the ultrasound machine and general principles for performing the scan.
- Patients should always have a short period of rest before scanning so as not to erroneously measure velocities in a hyperemic state.
- Specific features will be further discussed in the chapters covering diseases of different areas of the body.
- The principles for vascular tumors, malformations and fistulas are discussed in Chapter 12 and male genital studies in Chapter 14.

EXTRACRANIAL AND LOWER LIMB ARTERIAL STUDIES

Prepare the patient

- Read the referral and question the patient.
- Think about symptoms to predict the site of disease.
- Take a history and look for incisions for past operations such as a scar in the neck from carotid endarterectomy or scars in the leg from bypass grafting.
- For lower limb arterial studies, ask about the walking distance before onset of leg pain, where pain occurs, whether pain is relieved by rest and what else interferes with walking.

Select transducers – extracranial studies

- Use a medium- to high-frequency linear-array transducer for most extracranial studies.
- Use a curved-array transducer for a patient with a bull neck or to image the distal internal carotid artery.
- Use a phased-array transducer with its small footprint to study arch branches angling from above the clavicle medially and inferiorly, and the distal internal carotid artery.

Select transducers – lower limb arterial studies

- Use a medium- to high-frequency linear-array transducer for most arteries in the legs.
- Use a curved-array transducer for a patient with an edematous limb or who is obese, especially to image the superficial femoral artery at the adductor hiatus.
- Use a curved-array transducer if the tibioperoneal trunk or peroneal artery is difficult to scan due to heavy calcification or low flow.

Machine settings
B-mode
- Use the maximum dynamic range to aid plaque characterization.

Color Doppler
- Set the color velocity range to approximately +33 to −33 cm/s to highlight stenoses without spurious aliasing throughout the entire artery.
- Decrease the color scale and increase color gain to show low flow distal to an occlusion or high-grade stenosis.
- Choose a color map that easily highlights high velocities.
- Use a low wall filter setting to ensure that low velocities are not filtered out. Increase the wall filter to prevent wall motion artifact when scanning carotid arteries that are highly mobile with respiration.

Spectral Doppler
- Set the velocity scale to +130 to −30 cm/s.
- Use a small sample volume to help clear up the spectral trace.
- Place the sample volume in the center of the artery or within the stenotic jet stream.
- Decrease the spectral Doppler scale and increase spectral gain to show low flow distal to an occlusion or high-grade stenosis.
- Use a low wall filter to ensure that low velocities are not filtered out. Again increase the wall filter when interrogating highly mobile arteries.

Scanning techniques
B-mode
- Scan in B-mode in longitudinal and transverse to fully assess the arteries and plaque type.
- Locate arteries, stents and bypass grafts. These are easily differentiated from veins because they are mostly incompressible with transducer pressure.
- Orient arterial pathology to appropriate bony or vascular landmarks.
- Study atheromatous plaque in transverse and longitudinal with the color turned off to ensure correct characterization.
- Note the position and type of plaque, describe plaque morphology as homogeneous, heterogeneous or calcified, and describe surface characteristics as smooth, irregular or ulcerated.
- Measure diameters of arteries, aneurysms and grafts, and look for tortuosity or ectasia.

Color Doppler
- Take each artery in turn and use color Doppler to help identify the artery and highlight sites of increased velocities that indicate stenosis.
- Help identify arteries and bypass grafts.
- Note flow direction.
- Indicate the presence, location and length of each arterial stenosis or occlusion.
- Highlight areas of maximum velocities by color jets or color aliasing to show the best place to position the sample volume for spectral Doppler.
- Identify atheromatous plaque that is not visible with B-mode from a corresponding non-colored area in the color box.
- Identify collaterals and their flow direction.
- Identify the residual lumen diameter of an aneurysm.

Spectral Doppler

- Place spectral sample volumes to measure velocities at intervals along the artery, particularly proximal to, within and distal to areas of aliasing.
- Conclusively differentiate between arteries and veins by analysis of flow direction and waveform morphology.
- Determine which artery is being studied by whether there is a low- or high-resistance signal according to the particular arterial bed.
- Obtain a spectral trace of velocities proximal to and at sites of stenoses, and note whether spectral broadening is present or absent to help determine the severity of stenosis.
- 'Walk' the Doppler sample volume through a stenosis and use 'micromovements' from side to side to ensure that the sample volume is in the center of the artery or jet stream and that the highest velocities are obtained.
- Indicate proximal or distal disease from waveform analysis.
- Calculate appropriate ratios.
- Document the exact length and location of arterial stenoses and occlusions.

LOWER LIMB VENOUS STUDIES

Prepare the patient – venous reflux studies

- Ask about past deep vein thrombosis (DVT), pregnancies and previous varicose vein surgery and treatment.
- Ensure that there is sufficient light in the room to be able to see the varicose veins.
- Examine the leg for the site of varicosities to help predict connections for reflux.
- Medial thigh and calf varices suggest saphenofemoral junction (SFJ) incompetence, posterior calf varices suggest saphenopopliteal junction (SPJ) incompetence and localized 'bunches' may be due to incompetent perforators.
- Look for scars from surgery because this may be the only way to determine whether the great saphenous vein (GSV) or small saphenous vein (SSV) has been previously ligated or excised.
- Check to see if there are skin changes from lipodermatosclerosis, eczema or ulceration, and look to see where to avoid placing your hand for distal compression.
- Explain to the patient what is going to be done, particularly the Valsalva maneuver (see Chapter 11, page 206).

Prepare the patient – venous thrombosis studies

- Ask the patient for a history of DVT and to indicate the site of pain.
- The referring doctor may indicate whether iliac veins are to be scanned, but if not then a history and examination of pain or swelling in the thigh, recent pregnancy or past iliac DVT should persuade you to include iliac veins in the study.
- Warn the patient that compression is part of the test and can be uncomfortable or painful.
- Ask the patient to inform you when an area being compressed is particularly painful. This may indicate areas of thrombosis.
- Bowel gas can obscure abdominal scanning; fasting the patient before the examination helps to give a better view.

Select transducers
- Both deep and superficial veins are best imaged with a medium- to high-frequency linear-array transducer.
- A lower-frequency curved-array transducer may be required to scan an obese or edematous limb, deep veins in the thigh, particularly the femoral vein at the adductor hiatus, or peroneal veins.
- Curved- or phased-array transducers are required if the examination involves the inferior vena cava (IVC), or iliac, pelvic or ovarian veins.

Machine settings
B-mode
- Use low gain and power to prevent oversaturation of surrounding tissues or artifact within veins.
- High gain will cause thrombus to appear highly echogenic whereas low gain will better show low echogenicity.
- Use a high contrast setting (low dynamic range) to highlight vein walls when testing for vein compression or venous reflux.
- Use a low contrast setting (high dynamic range) to view thrombus and surrounding tissue.

Color Doppler
- Set a low color velocity range of +10 to −10 cm/s but increase the range if this produces unacceptably high color artifact or reduces the frame rate too much.
- Select a relatively even color hue across the frequency range because velocity information and aliasing are not used to test for venous disease.
- Optimize color gain and priority settings to allow good color filling without bleeding.

Spectral Doppler
- Set the velocity range to +100 to −100 cm/s when testing for reflux and +30 to −30 cm/s when testing for venous thrombosis. These ranges can be reduced for low-flow states.
- Set the wall filter to a minimum so that low flow traces are not filtered out.
- Open the sample volume to obtain as much information from the vessel as possible.
- Set the Doppler display sweep to the slowest speed to easily identify flow patterns.

Scanning techniques – all venous studies
- Venous scanning has less emphasis on spectral Doppler and more on B-mode and color Doppler.
- The sample volume does not need to be steered absolutely parallel to the vein wall.

B-mode
- Locate veins and map their course and connections.
- Identify perforators passing through the deep fascia.
- Measure diameters of incompetent saphenous junctions and refluxing saphenous veins and perforators.
- Assess whether veins can be compressed or contain visible thrombus.
- Classify the age of thrombus.

Color Doppler
- Distinguish veins from arteries.
- Show the direction of venous flow and indicate the presence of reflux.
- Determine whether the vein is patent, or partially or fully thrombosed.
- Identify collaterals.

Spectral Doppler
- Confirm venous occlusions.
- Confirm color Doppler directional information.
- Quantify duration of reverse flow to determine reflux.

Scanning techniques – venous reflux
- Take each vein in turn and identify it with B-mode in transverse.
- Then change to color Doppler to test for reflux in longitudinal.
- Use spectral Doppler with the sample volume filling the vein if there is doubt about the duration of reverse flow with color Doppler.
- Follow each vein along its full length with B-mode and periodically test for reflux with color Doppler.
- Detect perforators in transverse and test for reflux with the perforator 'opened up.'
- Use spectral Doppler if the color flow direction is ambiguous.

Scanning techniques – venous thrombosis
- Assess all veins for compressibility with B-mode in transverse. Use pressure from the transducer or counterpressure from the other hand to assess compressibility.
- Test for patency with color Doppler in longitudinal and transverse to ensure that a partial thrombus is not missed. This may be confirmed by spectral Doppler.
- Test for each at 1 to 2 cm intervals along the vein or when there is B-mode evidence of thrombus.
- Use spectral Doppler to test for phasicity in proximal veins. Reduced or absent phasicity indicates occlusion proximal to the test site.
- Sample a spectral trace from a vein to confirm loss of flow. If flow is seen throughout the veins then they are patent but may still be partially occluded.

UPPER LIMB VESSELS AND HEMODIALYSIS STUDIES

Prepare the patient
- Ensure adequate access to the neck and arms.
- Ask when symptoms occur and their nature.
- Explain the provocative positions to assess thoracic outlet syndrome and find out what position brings on symptoms.
- Feel for pulses.
- Ascertain location of arteriovenous fistula (AVF) or graft (AVG) from referral or patient's notes.
- Patients can also indicate location of an AVF or AVG.
- Feel for a palpable thrill over an AVF or AVG.
- Look for appearance of visible aneurysms over an AVF or AVG.

Select transducers

- A phased-array transducer with its small footprint is used for the suprasternal notch and to image deep vessels at the base of the neck.
- Use a medium-frequency linear-array transducer to image vessels from the shoulder to the elbow.
- A high-frequency linear transducer may be required for good images of vessels distal to the elbow or the superficial basilic and cephalic veins, or for a slim arm.
- A high-frequency linear transducer is needed to scan arteries for the Allen test and follow the superficial portion of an axillofemoral bypass graft.
- Use a high-frequency linear transducer to scan an AVF or AVG.
- A very-high-frequency hockey-stick transducer is suitable for digital arteries.

Machine settings and scanning techniques

- The principles for arterial scanning are identical to those discussed for carotid and lower limb arterial studies.
- For hemodialysis studies, set the color velocity range to +50 to −50 cm/s.
- The principles for venous thrombosis scanning are identical to those of the lower limb.

INTRA-ABDOMINAL STUDIES

Prepare the patient

- Read the referral and ask the patient relevant clinical questions.
- Take a history for past operations.
- For renal studies, a scar in the right or left iliac fossa may indicate the side of a renal transplant and a flank scar may indicate a nephrectomy.
- Diabetic patients should not fast.
- All other patients fast with the scan ideally performed in the morning.
- The following instructions for fasting are given:
  - For *24 hours* before the scan, avoid food and drinks known to produce gas such as carbonated drinks, beer and dairy products.
  - For *8 hours* before the scan, drink no more than small amounts of clear fluid. Cease smoking because this ingests air.
  - For *1 hour* before a scan for the kidneys, drink several large glasses of water.
  - Take your medications as normal with a little food if required.
- If a postprandial study is requested, give the patient a high-calorie, high-protein drink (flavored milk) and biscuits, and repeat scanning after 20 min.

TIPS!

- Apply reasonable pressure to the transducer to improve the image but not so much as to cause pain.
- Ask the patient to hold the breath while taking a Doppler sample; remember to tell the patient when to recommence breathing.

Select transducers

- Commence with a low-frequency curved-array transducer.
- Use the lower-frequency small-footprint phased-array transducer to allow angulation in several directions, including insonation beneath the xiphoid process or in the intercostal spaces, and to allow for bowel gas and large patients.
- A higher-frequency linear transducer is required to show a recanalized paraumbilical vein and liver surface or flow that is difficult to identify in the portal vein.

Machine settings

- Use high-gain settings for all modalities due to the depth of most vessels.
- However, high gain degrades spatial resolution so that there is a loss of contrast resolution if the signal is 'overgained.'
- In all modes, use zoom functions to interrogate regions of interest.

B-mode

- Use a high dynamic range (low contrast) to help visualize pathology such as mural thrombus in an aneurysm.
- Decrease sector width to increase the frame rate.
- Use only a single focal zone because multiple focal zones decrease the frame rate giving a blurred appearance.
- Scanning the liver effectively requires attention to optimization:
  - Set the depth only to the level of the deepest section of the liver.
  - Set the TGC to show even echogenicity throughout the liver.
  - Set the focus depth at the area of interest or, if examining the liver as a whole, set at its deepest surface.
- Compound imaging will improve edge definition of the liver surface.

Color Doppler

- Decrease the color box width to increase the frame rate.
- Use a medium to high wall filter because the abdomen moves with respiration causing wall motion artifact. Reduce the wall filter if no flow is detected.
- Set the color velocity range to approximately +33 to −33 cm/s to highlight arterial stenoses without spurious aliasing, or +10 to −10 cm/s for venous studies.
- Make sure that the beam is not approaching at too large an angle and that the velocity range and wall filter settings are not too high if a vessel can be seen but no flow is detected.

Spectral Doppler

- Increase the sweep speed when studying renal arteries because this allows better identification of waveform parameters required for criteria ratios.
- Set the velocity scale to +130 to −30 cm/s for arterial studies and +100 to −100 cm/s for venous studies.
- Use a low-to-medium wall filter.
- Sample a spectral signal from a vein to confirm loss of flow. If flow is seen throughout the veins, then they are patent although they could still be partially thrombosed.

Scanning techniques

- The principles for arterial examinations are identical to those previously discussed for carotid and lower limb arterial studies.
- Venous techniques are as previously described; however, when scanning for reflux no perforators should be present.

TIPS!

- It is difficult to produce intra-abdominal venous reflux using the Valsalva maneuver or distal compression.
- Abdominal venous reflux can be elicited by upper abdominal compression and arrested by lower abdominal compression.

4 EXTRACRANIAL CEREBROVASCULAR ARTERIAL DISEASES

Duplex ultrasound identifies the presence, severity and pathology of disease in extracranial arteries. Stroke is the third most common cause of death in western countries; about 75% are due to thromboembolism from extracranial arteries. Ultrasound is now used by many clinicians as the primary investigation to determine best treatment for extracranial arterial disease.

ANATOMY

Arteries scanned for reporting:
- Common carotid arteries – CCAs
- Internal carotid arteries – ICAs
- External carotid arteries – ECAs
- Vertebral arteries
- Innominate (brachiocephalic) artery
- Subclavian arteries.

Carotid arteries (Fig. 4.1)
- ECAs lie deep to the sternomastoid muscle.
- The CCA is medial to the internal jugular vein and vagus nerve.
- The carotid bifurcation is usually at the angle of the mandible.
- The ECA is anteromedial to the ICA at the bifurcation.
- The ICA is larger than the ECA.
- The ICA and CCA usually have no extracranial branches.

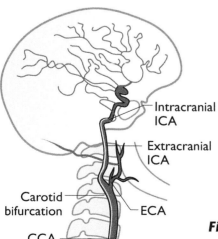

Fig. 4.1 *Extracranial carotid arteries.*
From Fig. 12.1c. Myers KA, Marshall RD, Freidin J. Principles of Pathology. Oxford: Blackwell, 1980. Reproduced with permission from Blackwell.

- The ECA has multiple branches. The first branch is the superior thyroid artery.
- The ICA may be looped or kinked.

Vertebral arteries (Fig. 4.2)
- They usually arise from the proximal subclavian arteries.
- They often differ in caliber.
- They lie lateral and posterior to the carotid arteries.
- Each passes to a canal in the cervical vertebrae, usually entering at C6 but higher in 5%.
- They enter the skull through the foramen magnum.
- They then join to form the basilar artery.

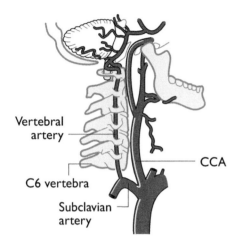

Fig. 4.2 *Vertebral arteries.*

From Fig. 10.2. Moore WS. Surgery for Cerebrovascular Disease. Philadelphia: WB Saunders, 1980. Reproduced with permission.

Aortic arch branches (Fig. 4.3)
- These are the innominate, subclavian and common carotid arteries.
- The innominate artery divides into the right subclavian artery and the right CCA.
- The left subclavian artery and the left CCA originate directly from the aortic arch.

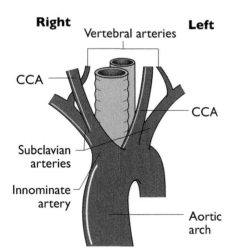

Fig. 4.3 *Aortic arch branches.*

Redrawn from Lord RSA. Surgery of Occlusive Cerebrovascular Disease. St Louis: CV Mosby, 1986. By kind permission of the author.

Abnormal origins from the arch (Fig. 4.4)

- Abnormal origins are not uncommon:
  - The innominate artery can supply the right subclavian artery and both CCAs (Fig. 4.4a).
  - There can be a common origin for the left subclavian artery and the left CCA (Fig. 4.4b).
  - Both subclavian arteries and both CCAs can arise independently (Fig. 4.4c).
  - The right subclavian artery can arise from the left side of the arch to pass in front of or behind the esophagus (dysphasia lusoria) (Fig. 4.4d).

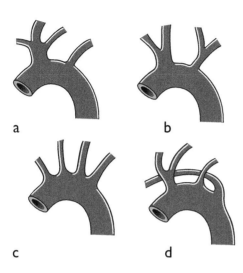

a

b

c

d

Fig. 4.4 *Abnormal origins from the arch.*

CLINICAL ASPECTS – ATHEROSCLEROTIC DISEASE

Regional pathology

Intima–media thickness and plaque

- Intima–media thickness (IMT) is a surrogate indicator for risk of arterial disease at any site.
- There is a strong correlation between IMT or early plaque and risk of future myocardial infarction or stroke.

ICA disease

- Stenosis usually occurs in the ICA bulb.
- Blood flow is not restricted until the lumen diameter is reduced by >50%.
- Symptoms usually result from ICA stenosis or occlusion.
- The risk of symptoms relates to the severity of stenosis and plaque characteristics.
- Cerebrovascular events are more often due to emboli from plaque than reduced flow from stenosis.
- Plaques that are echolucent or heterogeneous, or have intraplaque vascularity, are unstable and at greater risk of causing symptoms.
- Plaques with a large lipid core are very vulnerable.

ECA disease

- ECA stenosis or occlusion alone does not cause symptoms.
- ECA stenosis may contribute to cerebral ischemia if combined with ICA stenosis or occlusion.

Vertebral artery disease
- Stenosis commences at the origin.
- Thromboembolism can result from atherosclerosis at any level.
- Osteophytes can compress a vertebral artery in the cervical canal, often induced by turning the head.

Combined disease (Fig. 4.5)
- Carotid and arch branch disease may both be present as may extracranial and intracranial disease.

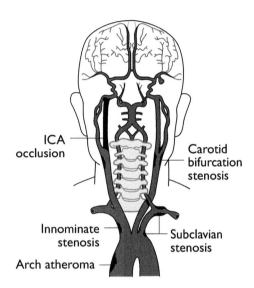

Fig. 4.5 *Common sites for extracranial arterial disease:*
- *The most common site is at the carotid bifurcation with plaque extending into the ICA, usually with a discrete end-point.*

Subclavian or innominate steal syndrome (Fig. 4.6)
- Subclavian or innominate artery disease can cause reversed ipsilateral vertebral artery flow to act as a collateral, to 'steal' blood flow from the brain to the upper extremity.
- The left subclavian artery is most commonly affected.

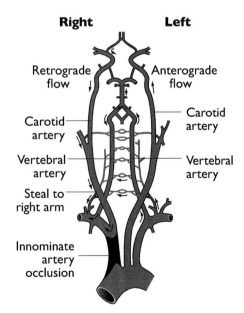

Fig. 4.6 *'Steal' from brain to right arm from innominate artery occlusion:*
- *Anterograde flow in the left vertebral and retrograde flow in the right vertebral artery.*
- *Reverse flow in the basilar artery.*
- *Flow through the circle of Willis to the basilar artery.*
- *Reverse flow in the right ICA and CCA.*

Clinical presentations
- Disease is most often asymptomatic.
- Transient or persisting symptoms with neurological deficit can be due to embolism or flow restriction caused by stenosis or occlusion.
- A cervical bruit can result from stenosis or tortuosity.

Symptomatic carotid territory disease
- *Transient ischemic attack (TIA)*: contralateral motor or sensory disturbance or speech impairment defined as lasting less than 24 hours
- *Amaurosis fugax*: transient ipsilateral monocular partial or complete loss of vision
- Stroke or blindness.

Vertebrobasilar insufficiency
- Visual disturbances and diplopia.
- Vertigo.
- Paraesthesiae.
- Impaired coordination.
- Drop attacks.
- Extrinsic vertebral artery compression possibly causing stereotypical symptoms.
- Thromboembolic ischemia usually causing persistent and varied symptoms which can proceed to a stroke.

Differential diagnosis
- Cerebral embolism from cardiac mural thrombus due to atherosclerotic heart disease or atrial myxoma.
- Cerebral embolism from thrombus or vegetations on heart valves due to atrial fibrillation, rheumatic heart disease, subacute bacterial endocarditis or mitral valve prolapse.
- Vasospasm of intracranial arteries from migraine or subarachnoid hemorrhage.
- Postural hypotension.
- Transient hypoglycemia.
- Inner-ear disease such as Ménière's* disease or middle-ear infection.

Treatment
- Severe ICA stenosis may require treatment by surgical carotid endarterectomy (CEA) or carotid artery stenting (CAS).
- Lesser degrees of disease are treated by medical measures.
- Past randomized trials have shown that CEA was superior to medical treatment for patients with >60–70% stenosis, but every clinician has a personal opinion as to the degree of stenosis that warrants intervention.
- ECA stenosis can be treated by surgical endarterectomy to improve cerebral perfusion if there is ICA occlusion.
- Vertebral artery endarterectomy or balloon dilatation may be performed for high-grade stenosis.

---

*Prosper Ménière, 1799–1862, French physician

WARNINGS!

- It can be difficult to distinguish tight stenosis from occlusion.
- A completely occluded ICA cannot be corrected by surgery and will not release emboli.
- However, very severe stenosis can be a potential source for emboli or acute thrombosis and may require urgent surgery.

CLINICAL ASPECTS – NON-ATHEROSCLEROTIC DISEASES

- Ultrasound may suggest a diagnosis but this almost invariably needs to be confirmed by arteriography and occasionally by arterial biopsy.

Regional pathology, presentations, and treatment

Fibromuscular dysplasia

- This usually involves the mid- to distal extracranial ICA on both sides.
- Presentation is with the same features as for atherosclerotic stenosis.
- Most patients do not require intervention but endovascular stenting is used if treatment is required.

Carotid artery dissection

- Dissection commences with a flap of intima and media from the ICA origin through the length of ICA, although it can start in the CCA or arch.
- Presentation is usually with a stroke.
- It is the most common cause of stroke in patients aged <45 years.
- Treatment is usually conservative with anticoagulation but endovascular stenting can be performed.

Carotid aneurysm

- This usually involves the distal CCA and proximal ICA.
- Arterial dilation is associated with mural thrombus.
- Presentation is with a pulsatile mass in the neck.
- Treatment is by resection with an interposition graft.

Carotid body tumor

- This is a highly vascular 'paraganglionoma' usually seen in the bifurcation between the ICA and ECA but sometimes higher to the base of skull.
- It is usually benign but can be malignant in 5% of cases.
- Presentation is with a mass in the neck which may be pulsatile.
- Treatment is by resection with an interposition graft.

Takayasu's ('pulseless') disease

- This usually causes occlusion or aneurysms of major arch branches.
- However, it can extend to more distal arteries.

- Presentation may be with cerebral ischemia or a pulsatile mass in the base of the neck.
- Treatment is by arterial bypass grafting.

Temporal (giant cell) arteritis

- Inflammation causes periadventitial edema.
- This affects the superficial temporal arteries in older females.
- Presentation is usually with severe headaches.
- Treatment is with steroids after which the ultrasound appearances typically disappear.

Moyamoya ('puffs of smoke') syndrome

- The condition affects children causing multiple occlusions or high-grade stenoses of extracranial carotid and vertebral arteries.
- Presentation is with cerebral ischemia.
- Treatment is by bypass of the superficial temporal artery to the middle cerebral artery.

WHAT DOCTORS NEED TO KNOW

- Is there atherosclerotic or non-atherosclerotic disease present?
- Which arteries are affected by disease and are they stenosed or occluded?
- What is the degree of carotid stenosis and the nature of the carotid plaques?
- Where is the carotid bifurcation and are there features that could make CEA more difficult – high bifurcation, tortuosity, coils and kinks, plaque extension or a narrow artery?
- What is the flow direction in the vertebral arteries and are they normal, stenosed, occluded or absent?
- Can aortic arch branches be seen and are they normal or diseased?
- Is the scan quality adequate to allow reliable management decisions without the need for arteriography?

THE DUPLEX SCAN

Abbreviations

- Peak systolic velocity (cm/s) – PSV
- End-diastolic velocity (cm/s) – EDV
- ICA/CCA PSV ratio
- Pansystolic spectral broadening – PSB.

Indications for scanning

- Lightheadedness, dizziness or non-specific visual disturbances – dubious indications for investigation.
- Cerebral territory symptoms.
- Vertebrobasilar insufficiency.
- Carotid bruit.
- Mass in the neck.
- Preoperative assessment before aortic aneurysm repair or coronary artery bypass grafting.
- Surveillance for patients with known stenosis treated conservatively.
- Intraoperative monitoring.
- Surveillance after CEA or stenting.

Normal findings

- *ICA*: a low-resistance signal because the brain is a low-resistance vascular bed. The PSV is <125 cm/s, there is a shallow upswing and the EDV is <40 cm/s.
- *ECA*: a high-resistance signal because it supplies a high-resistance vascular bed in the face. There is a sharp systolic upswing and low EDV.
- *CCA*: the signal is a combination of high- and low-resistance signals because flow passes to the two territories.
- *Vertebral artery*: PSV ≈ 40–60 cm/s with a low-resistance waveform because it supplies the brain.
- *Subclavian artery*: PSV ≈ 80–150 cm/s with a bi- or triphasic waveform and a prominent reverse component.

Criteria for diagnosing disease

Carotid intima–media thickness (IMT)

- Measured on the deeper wall of the CCA or ICA.
- Measured distance from the lumen–intima interface to the media–adventitia interface.
- Increases with age.
- Thicker in males than in females.

Carotid plaque characteristics

- Visual assessment of plaque echogenicity, texture and surface characteristics should be described, but is subjective and unreliable.

Surface
- Smooth
- Irregular
- Ulcerated.

Composition and echogenicity
- Homogeneous
- Heterogeneous
- Echolucent
- Echogenic
- Calcified.

ICA stenosis

- Grades of stenosis are based on criteria recommended by the American Society of Radiologists (Grant et al. 2003).*
- They recommended that all ICA examinations be performed with B-mode, color Doppler and spectral Doppler.
- ICA PSV and presence of plaque on B-mode and/or color Doppler images should be primarily used to diagnose and grade ICA stenosis.
- Two additional parameters, ICA/CCA PSV ratio and ICA EDV, may also be used when clinical or technical factors raise concern that ICA PSV may not represent the extent of the disease.

---

*Grant EG, Benson CB, Moneta GL, et al. Carotid artery stenosis: gray-scale and Doppler US diagnosis – Society of Radiologists in Ultrasound Consensus Conference. *Radiology* 2003;**229**:340–6

- Concerns can result for the following reasons:
  - ○ Discrepancy between the PSV and plaque appearance.
  - ○ Tandem lesions.
  - ○ Contralateral high-grade stenosis.
  - ○ Elevated CCA velocity such as with a hyperdynamic cardiac state.
  - ○ Low cardiac output causing generalized low velocities.
- The levels recommended for grades of ICA stenosis from PSVs and B-mode are shown in *Table 4.1*.
- The levels recommended for grades of ICA stenosis from EDVs and ICA/CCA ratios are shown in *Table 4.2*.
- An image for spectral analysis of a ≥70% stenosis is shown in *Fig. 4.7*.

Table 4.1 *Levels recommended for grades of ICA stenosis.*

Stenosis	PSV (cm/s)	B-mode and Doppler ultrasound
Normal	<125	No visible plaque or intimal thickening
<50% stenosis	<125	Visible plaque or intimal thickening
50–69% stenosis	125–230	Visible plaque
≥70% stenosis	>230	Visible plaque and lumen narrowing
Near occlusion	>230	Marked narrow lumen
Total occlusion	No flow	No detectable patent lumen

Table 4.2 *Levels recommended for grades of ICA stenosis from EDVs and ICA/CCA ratios.*

Stenosis	EDV (cm/s)	ICA/CCA PSV ratio
Normal	<40	<2
<50% stenosis	<40	<2
50–69% stenosis	40–100	2–4
≥70% stenosis	>100	>4

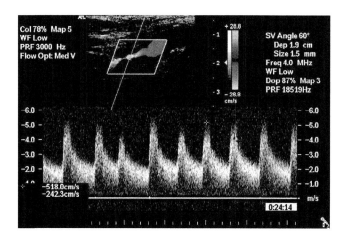

Fig. 4.7 *ICA spectral tracings for ≥70% stenosis.*

WARNING!

- Telephone the referring doctor if a symptomatic patient's scan shows severe ICA stenosis or ulcerated plaque (Fig. 4.8).

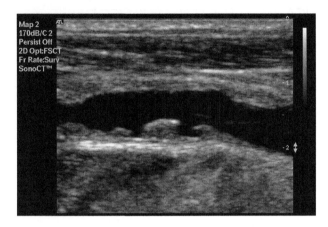

Fig. 4.8 *B-mode image of ulcerated ICA plaque.*

Image kindly supplied by Martin Necas, Hamilton, New Zealand.

CCA or ECA stenosis
- Criteria for CCA or ECA stenosis >50%:
  - PSV(distal)/PSV(proximal) >2.
  - Delayed systolic upstroke.
  - Post-stenotic turbulence and dampened distal signal.

ICA occlusion
- B-mode echoes from occlusive plaque and thrombus throughout the ICA.
- No color or spectral Doppler signal within the ICA.
- High-resistance CCA waveform with little, absent or reversed diastolic flow.
- Low-velocity, high-amplitude signal at the ICA origin – 'thump at the stump' (Fig. 4.9).

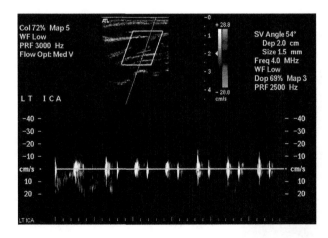

Fig. 4.9 *Spectral Doppler showing 'thump at the stump' for ICA occlusion.*

- Meniscus appearance of color Doppler at the ICA origin.
- Longitudinal pulsations rather than axial expansion of the occluded ICA.
- ICA narrowing making it difficult to image if the occlusion is long-standing.

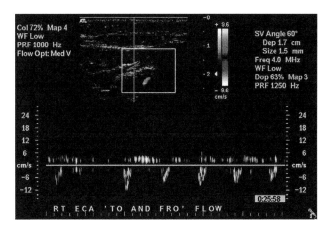

Fig. 4.10 *'To-and-fro' flow in the ECA passing to the ICA distal to occlusion of the CCA.*

CCA occlusion
- The full length is occluded and this may extend as an ICA occlusion.
- If the ICA and ECA are patent, there is retrograde or 'to-and-fro' flow in the proximal ECA (Fig. 4.10).

ECA occlusion
- This is usually segmental over 1–2 cm of the proximal ECA with a Doppler signal similar to an ICA signal distal to the occlusion.
- There may be reverse flow or 'to-and-fro' flow in proximal branches feeding the artery beyond the occlusion.

Intraoperative monitoring during CEA
- Ultrasound can be used in the operating theatre before completion of CEA to detect technical errors such as residual stenosis or intimal flaps, in order to revise the operation to reduce the risk of perioperative stroke or late restenosis.
- B-mode can detect technical problems causing hemodynamic abnormalities such as flaps, kinks or residual stenosis.
- Abnormalities in the ICA and CCA include raised ICA PSV >150 cm/s or ICA/CCA PSV ratio >3.0.
- Duplex scanning is more accurate than intraoperative angiography.

Postoperative surveillance after CEA or CAS
- Regular ultrasound scans can be performed to detect postoperative recurrent stenosis after CEA or CAS.
- However, criteria from PSV for severe restenosis are higher than those for unoperated disease, possibly because of greater stiffness in the wall.

- Criteria that have been shown to be appropriate when compared with angiography are (AbuRahma et al. 2008, 2009):*
  - CEA with Dacron patch:
    - >50% stenosis – PSV >215 cm/s
    - >75% stenosis – PSV >275 cm/s
  - Carotid stenting:
    - >50% stenosis – PSV >225 cm/s
    - >80% stenosis – PSV >325 cm/s

PITFALLS!

- Tortuosity:
  - This can cause apparent velocity increase even though there is no stenosis.
  - This is due to difficulty in obtaining a correct insonating angle, non-linear or helical flow, or increased velocity on the inside of the curve.
  - Try sampling just beyond the curve.
- 'Trickle flow' with low PSV caused by a very tight stenosis:
  - If flow is not detected, stenosis may be incorrectly diagnosed as occlusion.
  - Color Doppler can detect low flow with an ICA channel as narrow as the 'string sign' on arteriography.
  - Power Doppler or contrast imaging helps to detect low flow.
  - Apparent occlusion with ultrasound should be confirmed by arteriography, the reverse applies for apparent occlusion shown by arteriography.

Vertebral artery disease

- Criteria for >50% stenosis:
  - PSV ≥120 cm/s
  - (PSV − origin):(PSV − distal) >2
  - EDV ≥35
- A dampened signal suggests proximal vertebral artery disease and a high-resistance signal suggests distal disease.
- Vertebral artery occlusion can be confirmed only if a clear image of the artery is obtained.
- A high-grade ICA stenosis or occlusion can cause increased PSV and diameter in vertebral arteries because they act as collaterals through the circle of Willis.

Subclavian or innominate artery disease

- There are no established criteria for grading subclavian artery stenosis but it is reasonable to call it a stenosis if the PSV is >200 cm/s with post-stenotic turbulence and a distal dampened signal.
- Fig. 4.11 shows a typical spectral tracing in the vertebral artery when the ipsilateral subclavian artery is occluded.

*AbuRahma AF, Abu-Halimah S, Bensenhaver J, et al. Optimal carotid duplex velocity criteria for defining the severity of carotid in-stent restenosis. *J Vasc Surg* 2008;**48**:589–94

AbuRahma AF, Stone P, Deem S, et al. Proposed duplex velocity criteria for carotid restenosis following carotid endarterectomy with patch closure. *J Vasc Surg* 2009;**50**:286–91

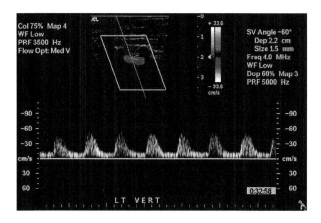

Fig. 4.11 *Reverse flow in a vertebral artery due to subclavian artery occlusion.*

Table 4.3 *Characteristic flow direction changes in extracranial arteries.*

Artery	Disease	R vertebral	L vertebral	R CCA	L CCA
	Normal	↑	↑	N	N
L subclavian	Stenosis	↑	↓, ↑↓ or ↑	N	N
L subclavian	Occlusion	↑	↓	N	N
R subclavian	Stenosis	↓, ↑↓ or ↑	↑	N	N
R subclavian	Occlusion	↓	↑	N	N
Innominate	Stenosis	↓, ↑↓ or ↑	↑	↑	↑ ↑
Innominate	Occlusion	↓	↑	↑	↑ ↑

↑ - anterograde flow; ↓ - retrograde flow; ↑↓ - to-and-fro flow; ↑ - decreased anterograde flow; ↑ ↑ - increased anterograde flow; L - left; N - normal flow; R - right.

● Characteristic flow direction changes in extracranial arteries with subclavian or innominate artery stenosis or occlusion (*Table 4.3*).

Fibromuscular dysplasia
● Ultrasound shows tortuosity and a '*string-of-beads*' appearance in the mid- to distal extracranial ICA (Fig. 4.12).
● Associated stenoses are present.

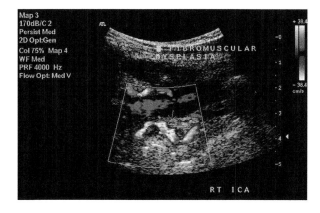

Fig. 4.12 *Color Doppler image of ICA fibromuscular dysplasia.*

Carotid artery dissection

- Ultrasound may show a long, narrow residual lumen through the length of the ICA or CCA or an ICA occlusion (Fig. 4.13).
- There may be visualization of an intimal flap.
- There is a limited sharp pulse due to relative obstruction (Fig. 4.14).

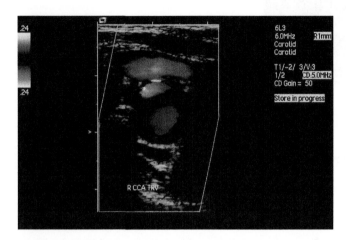

Fig. 4.13 *Transverse color Doppler image of CCA dissection.*

Image kindly supplied by Martin Necas, Hamilton, New Zealand.

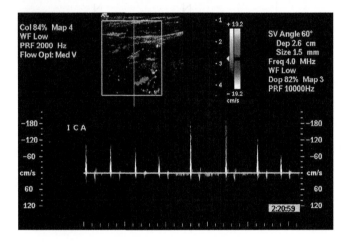

Fig. 4.14 *Spectral Doppler tracing of an ICA dissection.*

Carotid aneurysm

- Ultrasound shows that the dilation of the distal CCA and the proximal ICA is associated with mural thrombus.

Carotid body tumor

- B-mode shows a mass that splays the carotid bifurcation causing a 'saddle' appearance (Fig. 4.15).
- Color Doppler shows the tumor to be highly vascular fed by branches from the ECA.

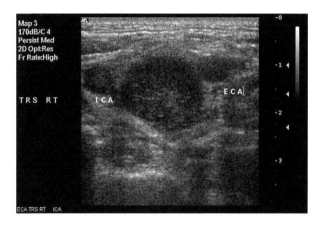

Fig. 4.15 *Transverse B-mode of carotid body tumor.*

Takayasu's ('pulseless') disease
- Characteristic ultrasound features are highly specific homogeneous circumferential intima–media thickening of the CCA on B-mode.
- There is reduced ICA flow and possibly reversed ECA flow on spectral Doppler.

Temporal (giant cell) arteritis
- Characteristic appearances are circumferential hypoechogenic homogeneous thickening of the superficial temporal artery wall.
- A characteristic 'halo' appearance is frequently seen on B-mode or color Doppler.

Moyamoya ('puffs of smoke') syndrome
- Ultrasound shows extensive arterial occlusions or high-grade stenoses of extracranial carotid and vertebral arteries with a rich collateral circulation.

PROTOCOLS FOR SCANNING
- Preparing the patient, selecting the best transducer, and general principles for scanning are discussed in Chapter 3 (pages 35–37).
- Always scan both sides.

NOTE!
- ICA disease can cause contralateral motor or sensory symptoms, or ipsilateral amaurosis fugax.

Carotid arteries
Position the patient and select windows
- Lay the patient supine if possible. Use one flat pillow or no pillow to extend the neck.
- Position yourself sitting either behind the patient's head or facing the patient.
- Turn the head 45° away from the side being examined with the chin tilted upwards.
- Vary the angle of approach or patient's head position as required.

- Move the transducer to where the arteries are most superficial.
- Image through the sternomastoid muscle with an anteromedial window or through the internal jugular vein with an anterolateral approach rather than through fat.
- Use a posteromedial window for the distal ICA to avoid interference by the mandible.
- Examine the carotid bifurcation from medial, anterior and posteromedial windows to find one that may counteract back-shadowing by calcified plaque.
- Use the submandibular window just below the angle of the jaw to show the more distal retromandibular extracranial ICA. This is useful to detect ICA dissections or fibromuscular dysplasia.

Scan the CCA, ICA, and ECA

- In B-mode, image carotid arteries in transverse from the clavicle to mandible with special attention to the carotid bifurcation, noting the relation of the ICA to the ECA. Note the position, extent and type of plaque and measure the diameters of the ICA, ECA and distal CCA.
- Use color Doppler to image the CCA, ICA and proximal ECA in longitudinal, noting areas of aliasing and lumen narrowing.
- Record spectral Doppler signals in the CCA, ICA and proximal ECA and any areas of suspected stenosis, noting the PSV, EDV and presence or absence of spectral broadening.
- Calculate the ICA/CCA PSV ratio.
- Note if there is tortuosity because this is a differential diagnosis for a bruit and is also important to record before a CEA.

TIPS!

- Disease is most common in the carotid bulb, so 'walk' a Doppler sample volume from the distal CCA through the proximal ICA to ensure detection of stenoses.
- Normal boundary layer separation within the carotid bulb is a reassuring sign that there is no stenosis.

Distinguish the ICA from ECA

- Image the arteries with B-mode:
  - ICA has a larger diameter than the ECA near the bifurcation.
  - ECA is anteromedial to the ICA at the bifurcation.
  - ICA usually then runs posterior to the ECA (but not always).
- Then image with color and spectral Doppler:
  - Use color Doppler to show that the artery with branches is the ECA.
  - Use spectral Doppler to show that the ICA has a low-resistance waveform (high EDV). and the ECA a high-resistance waveform (low EDV).
  - If in doubt, lightly tap the superficial temporal artery in front of the ear to produce a saw-tooth pattern in the ECA waveform; the tap test requires practice and the image should be interpreted with caution in inexperienced hands.

Distinguish severe stenosis from occlusion

- The aim is to detect trickle flow.
- Reduce the color velocity range to a minimum.

- Steer the color box straight.
- Use the venous scanning setup for low flow – low PRF and low wall filter.
- Increase color persistence.
- Reduce the angle of insonation.
- Use spectral Doppler because it is more sensitive than color Doppler.
- Increase the Doppler sample volume to cover the entire lumen.
- Change to a higher-frequency transducer.
- Consider power Doppler which is very sensitive to low flow.

Vertebral artery
Position the patient and select windows
- Straighten the patient's head and use an anterior or lateral approach.
- It can be difficult to see flow in vertebral arteries; if so then decrease the color scale, try different windows and turn the patient's head to the side.

Scan the vertebral artery
- Show the CCA and then find the vertebral artery just lateral and posterior identified by its path through dark 'shadowed' areas of the spinous processes.
- Use color Doppler to identify the vertebral artery.
- Vertebral arteries can be imaged from their origins to the mid-cervical region.
- Assess with spectral Doppler for flow direction and record PSV and type of resistance. What appears to be reverse flow may be due to tortuosity or flow in the adjacent vertebral vein.

Arch branches
Position the patient and select windows
- Turn the patient's head away from the side that you are scanning.
- Use the small-footprint phased-array transducer to angle over the clavicle if necessary.

Scan the subclavian and innominate arteries
- Examine each subclavian artery from its origin and record a spectral trace and PSV in a suspected stenosis.
- Plaque can often be seen using B-mode or a filling defect with color Doppler.
- Use color Doppler to highlight aliasing that indicates stenosis.
- Scan the innominate artery if stenosis is suspected.
- Record brachial systolic pressures in both arms if subclavian or innominate artery disease is suspected. A difference >20 mmHg shows that there is significant disease.

ULTRASOUND IMAGES TO RECORD
Atherosclerotic disease
- B-mode in longitudinal of the proximal and distal CCA, carotid bifurcation, and proximal ICA and ECA
- B-mode of significant plaque in transverse and longitudinal (color Doppler if plaque is echolucent)
- Sample spectral traces of the proximal and distal CCA, proximal and distal ICA, proximal ECA, and vertebral and subclavian arteries

- Spectral traces proximal to and at each stenosis; note the location from the anatomical landmark, severity and extent.
- Note the ICA/CCA PSV ratio.
- Spectral traces to confirm occlusion; note the location from the carotid bifurcation and extent.

Aneurysms
- Sample spectral traces in longitudinal for each artery listed.
- B-mode sample diameters for each artery listed.
- B-mode of length of aneurysm in longitudinal.
- B-mode of maximum transverse and anteroposterior diameters of aneurysm.
- B-mode of mural thrombus and residual lumen diameter of aneurysm.
- B-mode of proximal and distal diameters of adjacent normal artery.
- B-mode of distance of aneurysm for anatomical landmark.

Fibromuscular dysplasia
- Sample spectral traces in longitudinal for each artery listed.
- B-mode and color Doppler images in longitudinal, demonstrating the 'string-of-beads' appearance in ICA.
- Spectral traces proximal to, at and distal to areas of stenosis. Note the location from the carotid bifurcation, and the severity and extent of stenosis.

Carotid dissection
- Sample spectral traces in longitudinal for each artery listed.
- B-mode and color images demonstrating a false lumen in the affected carotid artery in longitudinal and transverse.
- B-mode measurement of length of dissection and location in relation to the carotid bifurcation.
- Sample spectral trace within false and true lumina.

Temporal arteritis and Takayasu's disease
- Sample spectral traces in longitudinal for each artery listed.
- B-mode longitudinal and transverse images demonstrating wall thickening and 'halo' appearance of affected artery.
- Spectral traces demonstrating occlusion or stenosis. Note the location from the anatomical landmark, and severity and extent.

Carotid body tumor
- Sample spectral traces in longitudinal for each artery listed.
- Transverse B-mode image of 'saddle' appearance of carotid bifurcation.
- Transverse color Doppler image of the carotid body tumor.
- Sample spectral trace in carotid body tumor flow.

WORKSHEET
Extracranial cerebrovascular arterial diseases

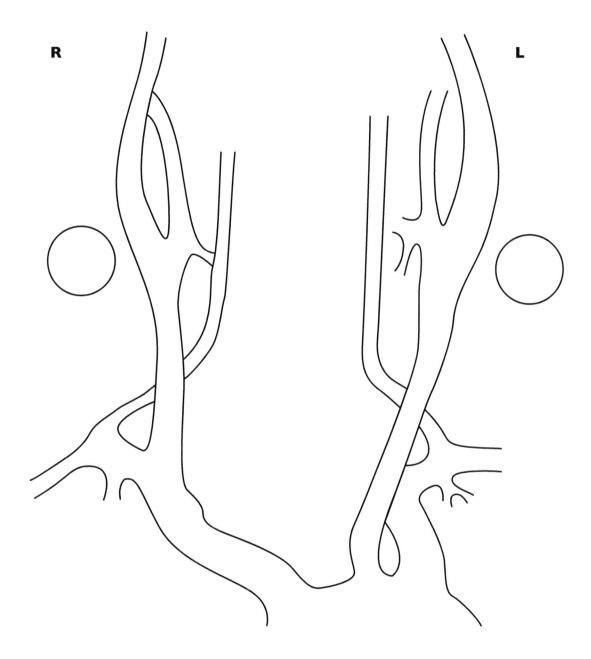

- Note PSV and EDV in the proximal ECA and subclavian arteries, proximal and distal CCA and ICA.
- Note flow direction in the vertebral arteries.
- Draw representation of plaque type and location, highlighting areas and degrees of stenoses.
- Draw representations of occlusions and their locations.
- Draw representation of proximal cross-sectional ICA plaque in the circles.

5 DISEASES OF VESSELS IN THE UPPER LIMBS

The most common indication for ultrasound assessment is to aid the diagnosis of the thoracic outlet syndrome. Arterial disease is less common in the upper than in the lower limbs and causes are more varied. Venous thrombosis occurs but venous reflux is rarely a clinical problem in upper limbs. Ultrasound is a good screening modality but many patients require digital subtraction angiography (DSA), computed tomography (CT) or magnetic resonance imaging (MRI) to help assess disease.

ANATOMY

Vessels scanned for reporting:
- Aortic arch
- Internal jugular vein – IJV
- Innominate (brachiocephalic) artery and veins
- Subclavian artery and vein
- Axillary artery and vein
- Brachial artery and veins
- Radial artery and veins
- Ulnar artery and veins
- Basilic and cephalic veins
- Dorsal arterial and venous arches
- Deep and superficial arterial and venous palmar arches
- Metacarpal arteries and veins
- Digital arteries and veins.

Other vessels discussed:
- Superior vena cava – SVC.

The thoracic outlet (Fig. 5.1)
- There are three consecutive spaces between the base of the neck and upper arm where compression of the brachial plexus (C5–T1 nerve roots), subclavian artery or subclavian vein can occur:
- The interscalene triangle is located at the base of the neck:
    - The boundaries are scalenus anterior in front, scalenus medius behind and the first rib at the base.
    - The lower brachial plexus and subclavian artery can be compressed because they lie behind scalenus anterior.
    - The subclavian vein cannot be compressed at this level because it lies in front of this muscle.
- The costoclavicular space is distal to the scalene triangle:
    - The boundaries are the clavicle, first rib, costoclavicular ligament and edge of scalenus medius.
    - This is the most common site for nerves, artery and vein to be compressed.

- The coracopectoral space is closest to the arm:
  - It is situated between pectoralis minor, the coracoid process, and the ribs.
  - This is the least likely space for compression to occur.

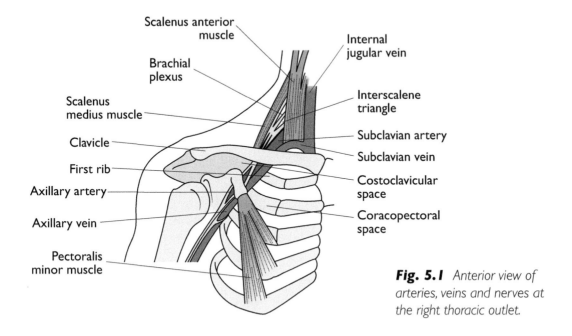

Fig. 5.1 *Anterior view of arteries, veins and nerves at the right thoracic outlet.*

Arteries at the thoracic outlet and axilla (Fig. 5.2)

- The innominate artery is the first branch of the aortic arch.
- The right subclavian artery from the innominate artery and the left subclavian artery from the aortic arch pass through the thoracic outlet.
- Each subclavian artery becomes the axillary artery as it passes from the thoracic outlet to the upper arm.

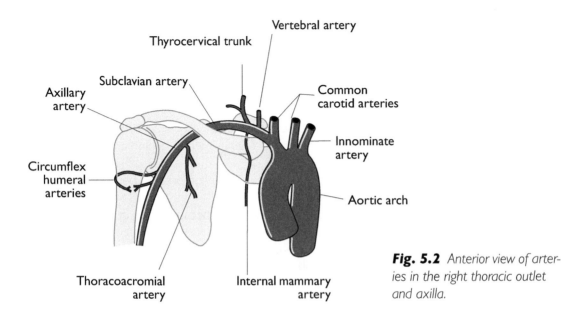

Fig. 5.2 *Anterior view of arteries in the right thoracic outlet and axilla.*

Arteries in the arm (Fig. 5.3)

● The axillary artery becomes the brachial artery passing to the elbow where it bifurcates.

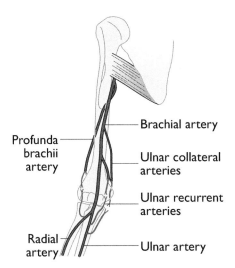

Fig. 5.3 *Anterior view of arteries in the right arm.*

Arteries in the forearm (Fig. 5.4)

● The radial artery is lateral and the ulnar artery medial, passing down to the hand.

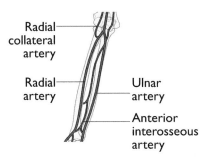

Fig. 5.4 *Anterior view of arteries in the right forearm.*

Arteries and veins in the hand (Fig. 5.5)

● At the wrist, the radial and ulnar arteries form each end of the dorsal and palmar arches.

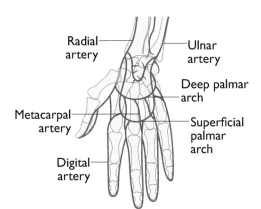

Fig. 5.5 *Anterior view of arteries in the palm of the hand and the fingers.*

- They each give a branch to form the dorsal arch on the back of the hand.
- The ulnar artery passes to the medial end of the superficial palmar arch and the radial artery to the lateral end of the deep palmar arch.
- Each artery then gives a branch to complete the two palmar arches.
- The deep palmar arch gives branches termed the metacarpal arteries which pass to the four fingers.
- These join with branches of the superficial palmar arch to form arteries which then divide to pass down each side of the four fingers as the digital arteries.
- The radial artery supplies the corresponding arteries to each side of the thumb.
- The dorsal venous network of the hand is formed by the dorsal metacarpal veins and continues up as the cephalic and basilic veins.

Veins in the neck and at the thoracic outlet and axilla (Fig. 5.6)
- The axillary vein passes through the thoracic outlet from the upper arm to the root of the neck to become the subclavian vein.
- The subclavian vein joins the internal jugular vein to form each innominate vein.
- The innominate veins join to become the superior vena cava (SVC).

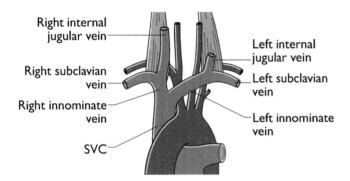

Fig. 5.6 Anterior view of deep veins in the neck, thoracic outlet and axilla.

Veins in the upper limb (Fig. 5.7)
- Superficial venous outflow is through the basilic and cephalic veins.
- The brachial, radial, and ulnar veins are paired.

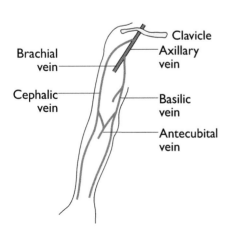

Fig. 5.7 Anterior view of venous outflow in the right arm.
- Deep venous drainage mirrors the arterial supply.

CLINICAL ASPECTS – THORACIC OUTLET SYNDROME

Etiology and regional pathology

- The subclavian artery, subclavian vein or brachial plexus can be compressed at the thoracic outlet (Fig. 5.8).
- The lower nerve roots are most often affected.
- Axillary/subclavian deep vein thrombosis (DVT) or severe obstruction: *Paget–Schrötter syndrome/effort thrombosis'* (Described by Sir James Paget in 1875 and Leopold von Schrötter in 1884.)
- Arterial compression can cause turbulent flow, post-stenotic dilatation, intimal disruption, aneurysm formation, thrombosis or embolism.
- Various bony or muscular abnormalities can cause thoracic outlet syndrome (TOS):
  - Cervical rib or its fibrous extension arises from C7 and passes to the first rib. It runs along the anterior border of scalenus medius immediately under the artery. It is present in <1% of individuals, 50% are bilateral and <10% cause symptoms.
  - Congenital abnormalities of the first rib are less common. The most frequent is first rib atresia leaving an exostosis on the second rib at scalenus anterior insertion.
  - Past fractured clavicle or first rib can impinge on the artery.
  - Fibrosis of scalenus anterior and scalenus medius can compress the neurovascular bundle where it passes through the interscalene triangle.
- Overuse of the arm due to work or sports activities can induce TOS, particularly in people with long necks and droopy shoulders.

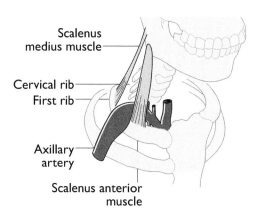

Scalenus medius muscle
Cervical rib
First rib
Axillary artery
Scalenus anterior muscle

Fig. 5.8 *Thoracic outlet syndrome: post-stenotic axillary artery aneurysm.*

Redrawn from Fig. 6.1, Myers KA. In: Chant ADB, Barros D'Sa AAB (eds), Emergency Vascular Practice, 1997. London: Hodder Arnold.

Clinical features

- Symptoms from nerve compression are more common than symptoms from vascular compression.
- The prevalence is difficult to determine due to uncertainty about the diagnosis in many patients with neurological symptoms.
- MRI studies show neurogenic TOS in 70%, venous TOS in 65% and arterial TOS in 40%, with frequent combinations of two or all three. Compression usually occurs in the costoclavicular space.
- Neurological features:
  - Pain around the shoulder and neck.
  - Referred pain, sensory disturbance or weakness down the arm.

- Venous features:
  - ○ Swelling, bluish discoloration and prominent surface veins in the arm and hand, made worse by strenuous physical activity.
- Arterial features:
  - ○ Arterial stenosis can cause coldness or vasospasm in the hand.
  - ○ Arterial occlusion or embolism can cause severe distal ischemia.
  - ○ Arterial aneurysm presents with a tender pulsatile mass in the neck.
- Examination for vascular compression from TOS by the 'military brace' maneuver (Fig. 5.9):
  - ○ It has a high incidence of false-positive results in normal individuals.
  - ○ A negative test virtually excludes vascular involvement.
  - ○ A positive test provides confidence to proceed with treatment if there is an appropriate history.

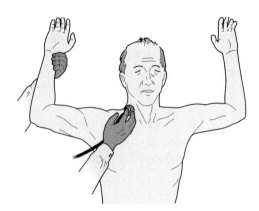

Fig. 5.9 *'Military brace' maneuver.*
Redrawn from Fig. 6.2, Myers KA. In: Chant ADB, Barros D'Sa AAB (eds), Emergency Vascular Practice, 1997. London: Hodder Arnold.

Treatment

- Neurogenic TOS is initially treated conservatively to improve posture and strengthen supportive muscles.
- Vascular TOS is usually treated by surgery:
  - ○ Removal of the first rib and cervical rib.
  - ○ Division of scalenus anterior and fibromuscular bands.
  - ○ Cervical sympathectomy may also be performed.
- Axillary/subclavian vein thrombosis
  - ○ Early detection: thrombolysis followed by vein balloon dilation or stenting.
  - ○ Delayed detection: anticoagulation as for deep vein thrombosis (DVT) in the lower extremities.
  - ○ Subsequent treatment: surgical decompression of the thoracic outlet.
- Arterial injury usually requires surgical repair with a bypass graft, although early cases can be treated by an endoluminal stent graft.

CLINICAL ASPECTS – INTRINSIC ARTERIAL DISEASES

Regional pathology
Atherosclerosis
- Disease can occur at any level.
- It is more common in the subclavian and axillary arteries than in more distal arteries.

- Proximal upper limb atherosclerosis frequently remains asymptomatic because of abundant collaterals around the shoulder.
- Severe innominate or subclavian artery disease can lead to reverse flow in the vertebral artery as a collateral to the arm for the 'subclavian steal syndrome' (see Chapter 4).
- Distal arteries may thrombose due to low-flow states.

Aneurysms
- Innominate or subclavian artery aneurysms are not uncommon.
- Most aneurysms are fusiform.

Autoimmune arteritis
- The following inflammatory arterial diseases can affect branches of the aortic arch to cause upper limb or cerebrovascular ischemia or more distal arteries to cause digital ischemia:
  - Takayasu's disease
  - Buerger's disease
  - Giant cell arteritis
  - Polyarteritis
  - Behçet's syndrome
  - Scleroderma
  - Hypersensitivity reaction
  - Systemic lupus erythematosus (SLE).

Other intrinsic diseases
- Fibromuscular dysplasia similar to that in the renal or carotid arteries has been reported in the brachial artery (see Chapter 4, page 55 and Chapter 7, page 126).
- Cystic adventitial necrosis similar to that in the popliteal artery has been reported in the brachial artery (see Chapter 6, page 102).

Clinical presentations
- Mild to moderate ischemia causing forearm fatigue or claudication.
- Severe ischemia leading to gangrene (Fig. 5.10).
- Palpable aneurysm.
- Raynaud's phenomenon.

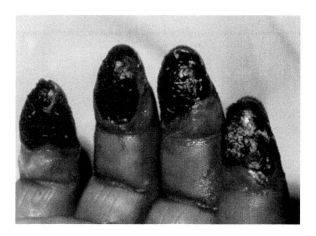

Fig. 5.10 Gangrene of the fingertips.

Treatment

- Surgical bypass (Figs 5.11 and 5.12) or endarterectomy may be required.
- Endovascular stenting or stent grafting are now widely used.

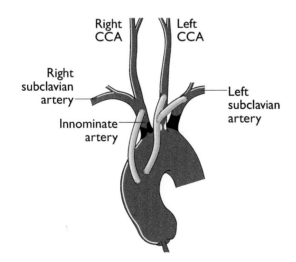

Fig. 5.11 *Transthoracic synthetic bypass grafting from the aorta to major branches. CCA – common carotid artery.*

Redrawn from Fig. 6.6, Myers KA. In: Chant ADB, Barros D'Sa AAB (eds), Emergency Vascular Practice, 1997. London: Hodder Arnold.

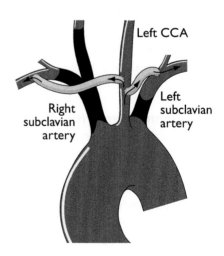

Fig. 5.12 *Extrathoracic common carotid to subclavian artery synthetic bypass. CCA – common carotid artery.*

Redrawn from Fig. 6.8, Myers KA. In: Chant ADB, Barros D'Sa AAB (eds), Emergency Vascular Practice, 1997. London: Hodder Arnold.

CLINICAL ASPECTS – OTHER VASCULAR DISORDERS

Etiology, regional pathology and treatment

Embolism

- Some 10–20% of emboli lodge in upper extremity arteries, most often in the brachial artery, less often the subclavian or axillary arteries and uncommonly arteries below the elbow.
- This may lead to consecutive thrombosis.
- The larger proportion comes from the heart but a third originate from innominate or subclavian artery disease.
- Embolism is treated by embolectomy through the brachial artery at the elbow.

Repetitive external trauma around the shoulder

- Throwing can cause injury to the axillary artery as a result of compression by the head of the humerus with the arm abducted and in external rotation.
- This has been studied in baseball pitchers, footballers and field athletes.

Repetitive external trauma to the hand and fingers

- Repetitive catching or striking a ball with the hand can cause digital artery or palmar arch thrombosis.

- *'Hypothenar hammer syndrome'* can occur in workers who hammer with their hands. The ulnar artery is damaged just beyond the canal under the hamate bone causing acute thrombosis or aneurysm formation.
- Treatment may require surgical repair or reconstruction.

Iatrogenic trauma
- Brachial artery catheterization for arteriography or hemodynamic monitoring.
- Venous catheterization for peripherally inserted central catheter (PICC) and central venous lines.
- Anesthetic arm block with accidental intramural injection.
- Thrombosed axillofemoral bypass.
- Arteritis after radiotherapy for carcinoma of the breast.
- Harvesting the radial artery for coronary artery bypass grafting if it is the dominant artery to the hand.
- Treatment is usually by surgical repair or reconstruction.

Venous thrombosis
- Upper limb DVT is usually due to TOS.
- Venous thrombosis from PICC or central venous lines.
- Thrombosis can result from a hypercoagulable state, but this is far less common in the arms than the legs, probably due to lower venous pressures and less venous stasis.
- The risk of pulmonary embolism from upper limb DVT is less than from the lower limbs.
- Treatment is with anticoagulation or with thrombolysis if detected early.

Raynaud's phenomenon*
- *Primary Raynaud's disease* results from vasospasm affecting the fingers due to abnormal sensitivity of the vasomotor nerve endings. Arteriolar spasm is induced by cold or emotional disturbance, particularly in young females.
- *Secondary Raynaud's syndrome* can result from many vascular conditions including the following:
  - Scleroderma: this can manifest as CREST syndrome:
    - C – calcinosis in the fingertips
    - R – Raynaud's phenomenon
    - E – esophageal dysfunction
    - S – sclerodactyly
    - T – telangiectasia
  - Thoracic outlet syndrome.
  - Atherosclerosis, arteritis or most of the arterial diseases discussed.
  - Connective tissue disorders such as rheumatoid arthritis or SLE.
  - Blood disorders such as abnormal cryoglobulins or cold agglutinins.
  - Use of vibrating tools to cause distal small artery vasospasm or occlusion leading to *'white finger syndrome'*.
  - Cold exposure.
  - Certain drugs.
- Unilateral Raynaud's phenomenon is always due to secondary Raynaud's syndrome.
- Treatment is for the underlying disease, vasodilator drugs, local care of the fingers, and cervical sympathectomy for severe cases.

---

*Auguste Gabriel Maurice Raynaud, 1834–1881, French physician

Clinical presentations

- Mild to moderate ischemia causing forearm fatigue or claudication.
- Severe ischemia leading to gangrene.
- Primary Raynaud's disease with color changes – pallor then cyanosis and rubor.
- Secondary Raynaud's syndrome causing trophic damage to the fingers or hands (Fig. 5.13).
- Microemboli or occlusive disease causing 'blue finger syndrome' (Fig. 5.14).
- Venous obstruction with arm swelling, edema, cyanosis, and visible collateral superficial veins.
- Difficult to infuse into or withdraw blood from a PICC or central venous line with pain along the vein and in the neck with arm swelling.

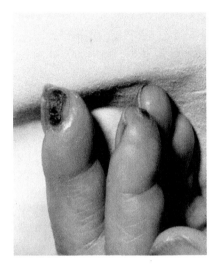

Fig. 5.13 *Trophic changes in the fingertips due to secondary Raynaud's syndrome.*

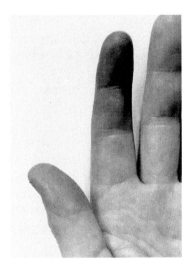

Fig. 5.14 *Blue finger from ischemia.*

WHAT DOCTORS NEED TO KNOW

- What is the pathology?
- Does it cause stenosis, occlusion, aneurysm or vasospasm?
- Are there spectral Doppler changes, B-mode evidence of vessel compression and fall in arm pressures with the 'military brace' maneuver to reveal TOS?
- Does mapping show a suitable size of the radial arteries for coronary bypass grafting?
- Which is the dominant artery to the hand before deciding whether to use the radial artery for coronary artery bypass graft (CABG)?
- Does mapping show suitable superficial veins for use as arterial bypass grafts?
- Is the PICC or central venous line surrounded by thrombus and what is its extent?
- Is there occlusive disease in the palmar arches, or metacarpal or digital arteries suggesting secondary Raynaud's syndrome?

THE DUPLEX SCAN

Abbreviations

- Peak systolic velocity (cm/s) – PSV
- Ratio of PSV at and just proximal to a stenosis – PSV ratio – V_2/V_1
- Pansystolic spectral broadening – PSB.

Indications for scanning

- TOS with arterial, venous or neurological features.
- Major arterial disease causing forearm claudication or hand ischemia.
- Raynaud's phenomenon causing hand ischemia.
- A pulsatile mass in the axilla.
- Arterial and venous mapping to select vessels suitable for a coronary artery or lower limb arterial bypass graft.
- Surveillance of an axillofemoral bypass graft.
- Arm swelling and pain or redness along an affected vein.
- Reduction in functionality of a PICC or central venous line.

Normal findings
Upper limb arteries

- Normal values for PSV are not well established.
- Probable representative PSVs are as follows:
  - Subclavian and axillary arteries – 70–120 cm/s
  - Brachial artery – 50–100 cm/s
  - Radial and ulnar arteries – 40–90 cm/s
  - Palmar and digital arteries – even lower PSVs.
- Normal waveforms are triphasic but peripheral resistance decreases with arm exercise or warming the limb and hand, causing the waveform to become monophasic with continuous flow through diastole.
- As skin temperature drops, waveforms remain triphasic but decrease in velocity.

Upper limb veins

- Deep inspiration increases venous flow.
- The Valsalva maneuver decreases venous flow.
- There is full color filling with distal augmentation.
- Pulsatile and phasic flow with respiration is seen in the internal jugular, innominate and subclavian veins (Fig. 5.15).
- Sudden sniffing causes momentary collapse of proximal veins and a brief increase in venous flow.
- Veins are compressible if they are accessible.

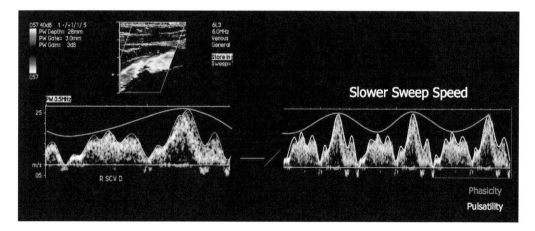

Fig. 5.15 *Spectral Doppler demonstrating phasic and pulsatile flow in a proximal upper limb vein.*

Image kindly supplied by Martin Necas, Hamilton, New Zealand.

Criteria for diagnosing TOS

- Increased PSV in the subclavian artery with the arm in provocative positions (Fig. 5.16).
- Extrinsic compression of the subclavian artery or vein with the arm in provocative positions.
- Dampened waveforms in the axillary artery with the arm in provocative positions.
- Arterial or venous dilation distal to extrinsic compression with the arm in provocative positions.
- PSB distal to extrinsic compression with the arm in provocative positions.
- 'Military brace' position causes pallor of the hand, loss of the radial pulse and a bruit at the base of the neck if the artery is compromised.

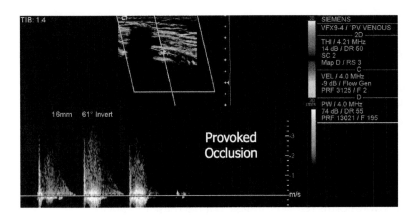

Fig. 5.16 Spectral Doppler demonstrating increased PSV, PSB and compression of the subclavian artery with TOS.

Image kindly supplied by Martin Necas, Hamilton, New Zealand.

Criteria for diagnosing upper limb arterial stenosis (Fig. 5.17)

- Criteria for upper limb arterial stenosis are not well established.
- PSV and PSV ratio criteria are generally assumed to be the same as for lower limb arteries (see Chapter 6, pages 107–108).
- Criteria to define subclavian stenosis are discussed in Chapter 4.
- With increasing degrees of stenosis, the waveform shows progressive PSB then post-stenotic turbulence.
- Dampened waveforms distal to high-grade stenosis.

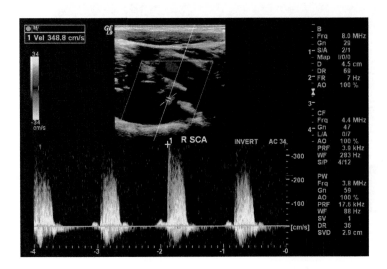

Fig. 5.17 Spectral Doppler demonstrating increased PSV and PSB due to subclavian artery origin stenosis.

Image kindly supplied by Martin Necas, Hamilton, New Zealand.

Plaque characteristics
- Composition and echogenicity:
  - Homogeneous
  - Heterogeneous
  - Calcified
  - Cauliflower calcified
  - Echogenic
  - Echolucent.
- Surface:
  - Smooth
  - Irregular.

Criteria for diagnosing upper limb arterial occlusion
- Occlusion is diagnosed with confidence if the following are observed:
  - No color Doppler or spectral signal in the occluded segment,
  - High-resistance spectral signal above the segment,
  - Low-amplitude spectral signal below the segment,
  - A collateral leaving the artery at the proximal end,
  - A collateral re-entering the artery at the distal end.

Criteria for diagnosing upper limb arterial aneurysm
- Maximum diameter is 1.5 times the diameter of the proximal diameter.

Criteria for diagnosing secondary Raynaud's syndrome
- Loss of color and spectral Doppler indicates occlusion in any segment of the deep and superficial palmar arches, and metacarpal and digital arteries.

Criteria for diagnosing axillofemoral bypass graft stenosis or occlusion
- Stenosis criteria are not well established, and are generally assumed to be the same for infrainguinal bypass grafts (see Chapter 6, page 108).
- Most departments use the PSV ratio to define significant graft stenosis with discriminant values reported from >1.5 to >3.0.
- A maximum PSV >350 cm/s or <45 cm/s also suggests imminent graft failure.
- Changes in the spectral waveform from tri- or biphasic to monophasic in the graft or inflow arteries indirectly predict graft stenosis.
- Occlusion is shown by lack of color and spectral Doppler throughout the graft.

Criteria for diagnosing upper limb venous thrombosis – direct evidence
Inability to compress the vein
- This is not a suitable criterion for innominate and subclavian veins because they cannot be compressed due to obstruction by ribs and clavicle.
- Thrombus prevents the vein walls from coming together with compression or during the sniff test for the subclavian vein.
- The vein can be partially compressed with partially occlusive thrombus but is incompressible with fully occlusive thrombus.

Intraluminal clot
- Fresh clot is echolucent whereas old thrombus is increasingly echogenic.
- This feature is highly dependent on image quality and instrument settings.

Absent flow in the vein

- There is no flow with occlusive thrombosis and only peripheral flow around a central non-occlusive thrombus.
- This is an important indicator for innominate and subclavian DVT where it is not possible to test for compressibility.

Diameter of the vein

- The diameter increases from the bulk of thrombus in the acute phase.
- It then gradually shrinks to become smaller than normal in the chronic phase.

Thickening of the vein wall

- The wall thickness gradually increases with time.

Criteria for diagnosing upper limb venous thrombosis – indirect evidence

Loss of phasic flow

- Diminished or loss of phasic flow with respiration (Fig. 5.18), or little or no response to the Valsalva maneuver in the proximal veins suggests obstruction proximal to the examination site.
- However, normal spectral Doppler cannot exclude DVT because there may be only partial thrombosis in more proximal veins.
- Of the criteria, this requires the most experience.

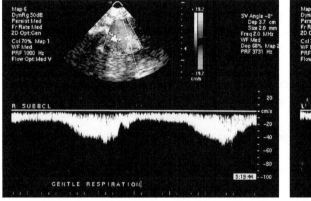 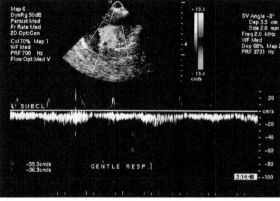

a   b

Fig. 5.18 *Phasicity with respiration shown with spectral Doppler in a subclavian vein:*
a *Phasicity with respiration in the normal left subclavian vein.*
b *Reduced phasicity with respiration distal to a partially thrombosed right subclavian vein.*

Loss of change of diameter with the sniff test

- No reduction of the subclavian vein diameter during the sniff test suggests thrombosis.

Minimal flow augmentation after distal arm compression

- This suggests occlusion between the examination and augmentation sites.

Increased diameter and flow in superficial veins

● The superficial chest wall veins enlarge if they are acting as collaterals.

Deep collaterals

● Large deep veins acting as collaterals may be seen adjacent to the thrombosed vein.

PROTOCOLS FOR SCANNING

● Preparing the patient, selecting the best transducer and general principles for scanning are discussed in Chapter 3 (pages 39–40).

Vessels in the thoracic outlet

Position the patient and select windows

● For proximal vessels, examine the patient seated or standing so that the shoulder girdle is relaxed and falls down under gravity to improve access.
● Examine subclavian and axillary vessels through suprasternal, supraclavicular and infraclavicular windows.
● Use copious gel to maintain good skin contact in the suprasternal notch.
● The axillary artery is easier to see with the arm abducted and scanned from an axillary approach, but it can be scanned through an anterior window.
● Provocative positions for the TOS:
  ○ 'Military brace' position:
    ● Arms elevated to 90° with the shoulders forced back as far as possible.
    ● Opening and closing the hands 20 times.
  ○ Adson's maneuver:
    ● Arms dependent.
    ● Neck braced backwards and head turned to the ipsilateral side.
    ● Patient holding in a deep breath.
  ○ Abduction to 90° or 180°.
  ○ Any position that brings on symptoms.
● Examine the IJV with the patient supine to distend the vein walls.

NOTE!

● If there is excessive movement of vessels with respiration, ask the patient to hold his or her breath; do not forget to tell him or her when to breathe again.

PITFALL!

● Scanning upper limb vessels can be challenging due to variations in anatomy and difficulties in negotiating the clavicle.

Upper limb vessels beyond the thoracic outlet
Position the patient and select windows

- With the patient upright or lying supine, externally rotate the arm to view the brachial vessels from a medial window between triceps and biceps.
- It is easier to scan with the patient supine with the arm externally rotated for the vessels of the forearm.
- For veins, the patient may be seated or standing in order to fill the veins for better identification.

Scan for TOS

- Use color Doppler to identify the proximal subclavian artery and highlight areas of color aliasing. Record a sample spectral trace.
- Take sample spectral traces and record PSV proximal to, at and distal to sites of stenosis to classify the severity, extent and location from an anatomical landmark.
- Take sample spectral traces proximal to, within and distal to occlusions to demonstrate the extent and location from an anatomical landmark.
- If a tight stenosis or occlusion is present in the subclavian artery, examine the ipsilateral vertebral artery for reverse flow.
- If monophasic or dampened waveforms are present in the proximal subclavian artery, investigate the innominate artery if on the right side or, if possible, the distal aortic arch for the left side.
- With the arm at rest, use B-mode to measure the lumen diameter of the subclavian artery and vein just proximal and distal to the clavicle.
- With the arm at rest, record sample spectral traces in the subclavian artery and vein just proximal and distal to the clavicle, and within the proximal axillary artery and vein.
- With the arm in the previously mentioned provocative positions, repeat the above two sets of measurements.
- Note if there is arterial or venous aneurysmal dilation distal to extrinsic compression at the level of the clavicle.
- If an aneurysm is present, use B-mode to measure its proximal, maximum and distal diameters.
- Note the presence of mural thrombus and record residual diameter.

NOTE!

- **Examine both arms for TOS even if there are only unilateral symptoms.**

Scan for arterial disease

- Use color Doppler to identify the proximal subclavian artery and highlight areas of color aliasing. Record a sample spectral trace.
- If stenosis is present, record PSV proximal to, at and distal to sites of stenosis, and classify the severity, extent and location from an anatomical landmark.
- Record spectral traces proximal to, within and distal to an occlusion, and measure its location and length.
- If a tight stenosis or occlusion is present in the subclavian artery, examine the ipsilateral vertebral artery for reverse flow.

- If monophasic or dampened waveforms are present in the proximal subclavian artery, investigate the innominate artery if on the right side or, if possible, the distal aortic arch for the left side.
- Follow the upper limb arteries in longitudinal with color Doppler to highlight areas of color aliasing, and use spectral Doppler to obtain sample spectral traces.
- If stenosis is present, record PSV proximal to, at and distal to sites of stenosis, and classify the severity, location, and extent.
- Record spectral traces proximal to, within and distal to an occlusion to demonstrate extent and location from an anatomical landmark.
- Note location of stenosis or occlusion measured from the elbow or wrist.
- PSV progressively falls the more distally you scan, so continually decrease the color scale to ensure adequate color filling.
- The radial artery is a more direct extension of the brachial artery than the ulnar artery.
- If thrombus is thought to be seen in distal arteries, the axillary, subclavian and brachial arteries must be scanned for aneurysms containing mural thrombus.
- Use B-mode in transverse to measure representative normal diameters.
- If an aneurysm is present, use B-mode to measure its proximal, maximum and distal diameters.
- Note the presence of mural thrombus and record the residual diameter. Note length and location from an anatomical landmark.
- If Raynaud's syndrome is to be investigated, continue distally, scanning the deep and superficial palmar arches, metacarpal and digital arteries.

Scan for venous thrombosis

- Image the internal jugular veins from the base of the neck to as high as possible in transverse, using B-mode to test for compressibility, and spectral and color Doppler to test for spontaneous color filling, pulsatile flow and respiratory fluctuations.
- Have the patient perform the sniff test to see if the innominate and subclavian veins collapse, indicating that they are thrombus free.
- Examine the subclavian and axillary veins in longitudinal and spectral Doppler to assess flow patterns with respiration and the Valsalva maneuver.
- Examine the axillary vein in B-mode and transverse to see if it is dilated due to proximal compression at the level of the clavicle.
- Scan the axillary, brachial, radial and ulnar, and cephalic and basilic veins for fully and partially occlusive thrombus.
- Use color Doppler to look for color filling defects, spectral Doppler to confirm loss of venous flow and B-mode for compressibility.
- Use color Doppler at 1- to 2-cm intervals to show vein patency by augmentation after distal arm or forearm compression.
- If thrombus is present, measure extent and location from an anatomical landmark.
- If indicated, follow the PICC or central venous line from its insertion to its proximal extent, testing for thrombus.

NOTE!

- Incompetence studies are not performed because upper limb varicose veins are rare.

Scan for radial artery harvesting pre-CABG

- Record PSV and note direction of flow in the radial aspect of the superficial palmar arch before and after compression of the radial artery, as for the Allen test (see below). This region is located in the crease of the proximal palm at the base of the thumb.
- If the Allen test is negative, scan the radial artery for atherosclerotic disease to assure suitability for harvesting.
- Also scan the ulnar artery for atherosclerotic disease because a diseased artery may not supply adequate hand perfusion post-radial artery harvest.
- Take sample spectral traces for the radial and ulnar arteries and, if stenosis is present, record PSV proximal to, at and distal to sites of stenosis, and classify the severity, extent and location from an anatomical landmark.
- In transverse B-mode, measure the diameter of the lumen in the proximal, mid and distal radial artery.

Scan for venous harvesting pre-femoropopliteal bypass graft

- Use B-mode to determine patency, lumen diameter and sites of communication with perforators and tributaries of the cephalic and basilic veins.
- Use B-mode for compression testing, and color Doppler with distal augmentation to detect thrombus or wall thickening in veins.
- Use spectral Doppler to confirm color Doppler findings.

Scan for axillofemoral bypass graft

- Find the proximal anastomosis using B-mode and color Doppler.
- Look for regions of inflow stenosis proximal to and at the proximal anastomosis.
- In B-mode, examine the proximal anastomosis for an aneurysm.
- If aneurysm is present, use B-mode to measure maximum diameters, proximal native artery and proximal graft diameters.
- Use color Doppler in longitudinal to follow the graft to its distal anastomosis, looking for regions of stenosis indicated by color aliasing.
- Record sample spectral traces from the proximal, mid and distal graft, and record PSV proximal to, at and distal to sites of stenosis to classify their severity, extent and location in relation to the graft origin.
- Examine the distal anastomosis for aneurysm and stenosis.
- Examine distal outflow for stenosis and patency.
- Examine the graft for incorporation into surrounding tissues or perigraft collection.

OTHER INVESTIGATIONS

The Allen test*

- This is a clinical test observing color changes to determine the distribution of occlusive arterial disease in the hands and fingers.
- Continuous-wave Doppler, photoplethysmography or duplex ultrasound can be used to supplement clinical observation.
- Presence of flow and direction are observed in the radial and ulnar arteries in the hand, distal to active compression of each artery in turn at the wrist.
- The technique is as follows (Fig. 5.19):
  ○ With the arm slightly raised, the radial and ulnar arteries are compressed and the hand is exercised to produce ischemia (Fig. 5.19a).

---

*Edgar Van Nuys Allen, 1900–1961, American physician

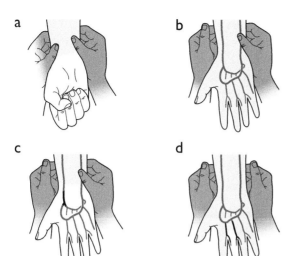

Fig. 5.19 *The Allen test.*

Redrawn from Fig. 6.3, Myers KA. In: Chant ADB, Barros D'Sa AAB (eds), Emergency Vascular Practice, 1997. London: Hodder Arnold.

- ○ Normal finding – compression of one or both arteries is released and there is prompt reactive hyperemia of the hand (Fig. 5.19b).
- ○ Radial artery occlusion – radial artery compression is released but there is no immediate reactive hyperemia (Fig. 5.19c).
- ○ Ulnar artery occlusion – ulnar artery compression is released but there is no immediate reactive hyperemia.
- ○ Metacarpal artery occlusions – arterial compression is released and all fingers show reactive hyperemia except the finger affected by disease (Fig. 5.19d).
- The aims are as follows:
  - ○ To detect occlusive arterial disease in the radial or ulnar artery, or the palmar arches and their branches, particularly with secondary Raynaud's syndrome.
  - ○ To determine whether the radial or ulnar artery is the dominant artery to the hand before deciding whether to use the radial artery as a bypass graft to ensure that its removal does not cause hand ischemia.

Pressure measurements
- Use continuous-wave Doppler to measure systolic pressures in the brachial, radial and ulnar arteries after deflating a sphygmomanometer cuff.
- A pressure difference >20 mmHg between sides at the same level indicates occlusive disease in the side with the lowest pressure.
- As with lower limbs, heavily calcified arteries can cause spuriously high pressure readings.

ULTRASOUND IMAGES TO RECORD
TOS
- Sample spectral trace in the proximal subclavian artery.
- Spectral traces proximal to, at, and distal to each stenosis; note location, extent, and severity.
- B-mode of plaques in longitudinal.
- Sample spectral traces in the subclavian artery just proximal and distal to the clavicle and within the axillary artery at rest, and with the arm in different provocative positions.

- Spectral trace in regions of extrinsic compression.
- B-mode of diameters of the subclavian artery just proximal and distal to the clavicle and within the axillary artery at rest, and with the arm in different provocative positions.
- B-mode of diameter in region of extrinsic compression of subclavian artery.
- Sample spectral traces in the subclavian vein just proximal and distal to the clavicle and within the axillary vein at rest, with the Valsalva maneuver, distal augmentation and the arm in different provocative positions.
- B-mode of diameters of the subclavian vein just proximal and distal to the clavicle and within the axillary vein at rest, and with the arm in different provocative positions.
- B-mode of diameter in region of extrinsic compression of subclavian vein.

Atherosclerotic disease and graft surveillance

- Sample spectral traces in longitudinal for each artery listed.
- Sample spectral traces in the artery above and below a bypass graft and in the proximal, mid and distal graft.
- Spectral traces proximal to, at and distal to each stenosis.
- Note the location from an anatomical landmark, the extent and the severity.
- Spectral traces proximal to, within and distal to occlusions; note the location from an anatomical landmark and the extent.
- B-mode of plaques in longitudinal.

Aneurysms

- B-mode of length of aneurysm in longitudinal.
- B-mode of maximum diameters of aneurysm.
- B-mode of mural thrombus and residual lumen diameter of aneurysm.
- B-mode of proximal and distal diameters of adjacent normal artery.

Venous thrombosis

- Transverse B-mode dual images to demonstrate compressibility of all appropriate superficial and deep veins of the arm.
- Sample spectral trace in longitudinal for flow in the proximal veins with normal respiration and the Valsalva maneuver.
- B-mode in longitudinal of the subclavian artery during the sniff test.
- Sample spectral trace of all mid to distal veins during distal augmentation.
- Spectral trace and color Doppler images to demonstrate lack of flow in thrombosed veins.
- Note the extent and location of thrombus to an anatomical landmark.
- Note whether thrombus is occlusive or non-occlusive and whether recanalization is present.

Radial artery harvesting pre-CABG

- Sample spectral traces of radial side of superficial palmar arch with the radial artery compressed and non-compressed; note directions of flow.
- Transverse B-mode diameters of inner lumen of proximal, mid and distal radial artery.
- B-mode images of radial and ulnar artery disease.
- Sample spectral trace of radial and ulnar arteries.
- Spectral traces proximal to, at and distal to each stenosis; note the location from the anatomical landmark, the extent and the severity.

Venous harvesting pre-femoropopliteal bypass graft

- Transverse B-mode dual images to demonstrate compressibility of the cephalic and basilic veins.
- Color Doppler images with distal augmentation to demonstrate thrombus or wall thickening.
- B-mode image of thrombus; note the location and extent from an anatomical landmark.
- Transverse B-mode images of representative lumen diameters.
- Note the location of communication with perforators and large tributaries from the anatomical landmark.

Axillofemoral bypass graft

- Sample spectral traces in the artery above and below a bypass graft and in the proximal, mid and distal graft.
- B-mode diameters of any aneurysmal dilation at anastomosis sites and within the native artery and unaffected adjacent graft.
- Spectral traces proximal to, at and distal to each stenosis; note the location from the anatomical landmark, the extent and the severity.
- Spectral trace within occluded graft.
- B-mode image of any perigraft collections.

WORKSHEET
Upper limb arterial

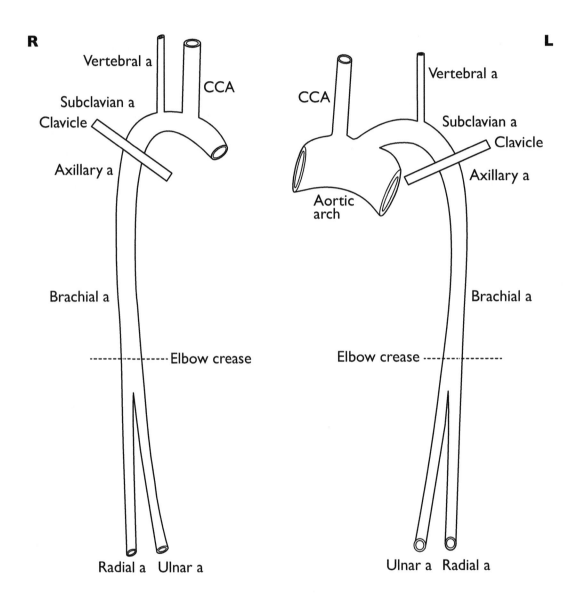

- Draw representation of plaque type and location, highlighting areas and degrees of stenoses.
- Draw representations of occlusions and their locations.

WORKSHEET
Upper limb venous

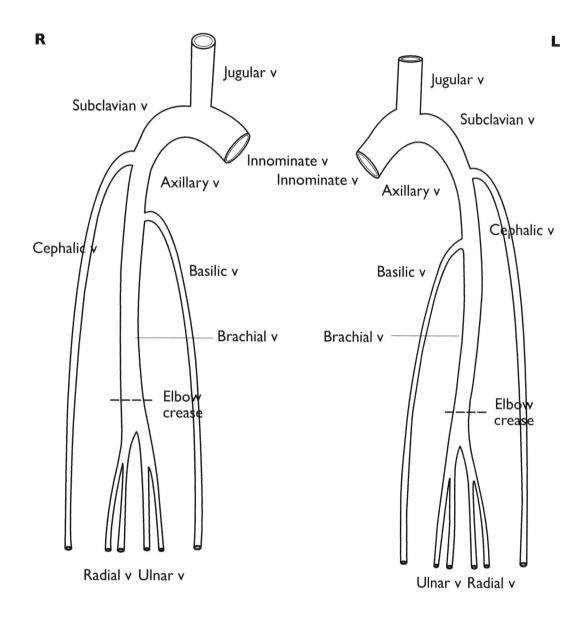

- Draw representation of thrombus and location.

DISEASES OF ARTERIES TO THE LOWER LIMBS

Duplex scanning can determine the location, extent and type of occlusive or aneurysmal disease. Ultrasound is commonly used to plan clinical treatment for occlusive disease, followed by arteriography if intervention is required. Ultrasound is used for screening and surveillance of aneurysms, but computed tomography (CT) more accurately measures size whereas arteriography is required in selected patients.

ANATOMY

Arteries scanned for reporting:
- Abdominal aorta
- Common iliac artery – CIA
- Internal iliac artery – IIA
- External iliac artery – EIA
- Common femoral artery – CFA
- Profunda femoris artery – PFA
- Superficial femoral artery – SFA
- Popliteal artery
- Tibioperoneal trunk – TPT
- Posterior tibial artery – PTA
- Anterior tibial artery – ATA
- Peroneal artery.

Abdominal aorta (Fig. 6.1)
- Lies to the left of the midline with the inferior vena cava (IVC) to its right.
- Extends from L1 to L4 vertebrae.

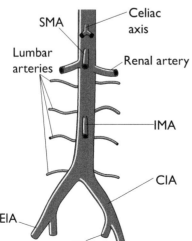

Fig. 6.1 *Anterior view of abdominal aorta. (SMA – superior mesenteric artery; IMA – inferior mesenteric artery).*

- Gives visceral branches.
- Gives phrenic and lumbar parietal branches.
- Divides into the common iliac arteries at the level of the umbilicus.

CIA (Fig. 6.2)
- Extends from L4 to the sacroiliac joint.
- Approximately 4–5 cm long.
- Divides into the IIA and EIA.
- Lies to the left of the corresponding common iliac vein (CIV).

IIA (Fig. 6.2)
- Splits into anterior and posterior divisions.
- The anterior division gives branches that supply the reproductive organs, bladder, rectum and buttock.
- The posterior division gives branches to the pelvic muscles.

EIA (Fig. 6.2)
- Approximately twice the length of the CIA.
- Lies superficial to the corresponding vein.
- Gives an inferior epigastric artery passing upwards and anterior just above the inguinal ligament.
- Becomes the CFA at the inguinal ligament.
- May bifurcate into the SFA and PFA (rare).

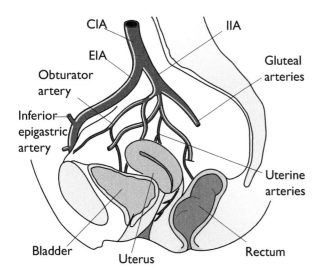

Fig. 6.2 *Oblique view of right iliac arteries (female).*

CFA (Fig. 6.3)
- Lies superficial in the femoral triangle below the inguinal ligament.
- Extends for 3–5 cm beyond the inguinal ligament.
- Divides to form the SFA and PFA.
- Ascending branches that anastomose with IIA branches are the superficial and deep external pudendal, superficial epigastric and superficial circumflex iliac arteries.
- Descending branch is the descending genicular artery.
- May be absent with a bifurcation above the inguinal ligament (rare).

PFA (Fig. 6.3)

- Provides lateral and medial circumflex femoral arteries.
- Gives perforating arteries to thigh muscles.

SFA (Fig. 6.3)

- Extends down the medial thigh.
- Passes deep through the hiatus of adductor magnus.

Popliteal artery (Figs 6.3 and 6.4)

- Commences beyond the adductor hiatus.
- Passes vertically through the popliteal fossa.
- Divides to form the TPT and the ATA.

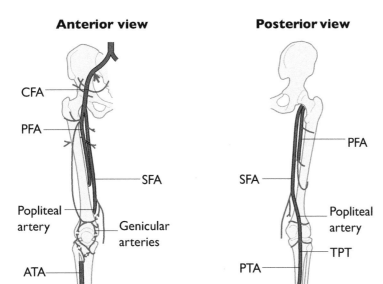

Fig. 6.3 *Anterior and posterior views of right femoral and popliteal arteries.*

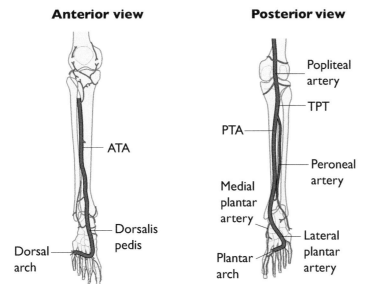

Fig. 6.4 *Anterior and posterior views of right infrapopliteal arteries.*

Infrapopliteal arteries (Fig. 6.4)

- These consist of the tibioperoneal trunk, ATA, PTA and peroneal arteries.
- The tibioperoneal trunk divides to form the PTA and peroneal artery.
- The ATA passes anterior to the tibia to supply the anterior compartment and continues as the dorsalis pedis artery in the foot.
- The PTA runs posterior to the tibia to supply the back of the calf and continues as the plantar arteries in the foot.
- The peroneal artery runs medial to the fibula to supply the deep compartment.
- There are several interconnections so that each can supply all regions.

CLINICAL ASPECTS – ATHEROSCLEROTIC OCCLUSIVE DISEASE

Regional pathology

Extent of disease

- Disease is segmental rather than diffuse.
- Stenoses result from atheromatous plaques (Fig. 6.5).
- Occlusions result from secondary thrombosis between branches that supply collaterals.
- Proximal occlusions usually affect the full length of the infrarenal aorta or the CIA or EIA because each usually has small or no branches (Fig. 6.6).
- Infrainguinal occlusions can affect the SFA between two large muscular branches, or the popliteal artery and infrapopliteal arteries (Fig. 6.7).
- There may be multiple occlusions with isolated patent segments between (Fig. 6.8).

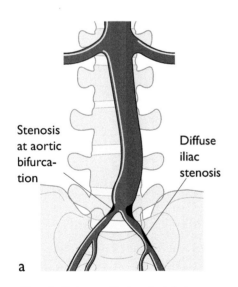
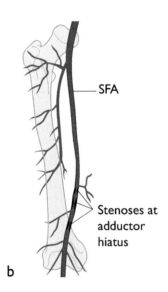

Fig. 6.5 *Lower limb arterial stenoses.*

- *Common sites:*
- **a** *Aortic bifurcation extending through the iliac arteries.*
- **b** *SFA at the adductor hiatus.*

Reproduced from Fig. 12.1 e,f, Myers KA, Marshall RD, Freidin J. Principles of Pathology. Oxford: Blackwell, 1980 with permission from Blackwell.

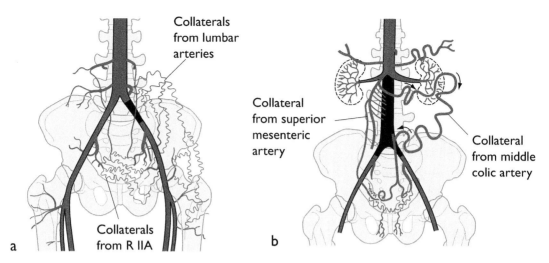

Fig. 6.6 *Aortic and iliac artery occlusions.*
a CIA occlusion; collaterals:
- *Arise from parietal arteries,*
- *Pass to IIA and PFA branches.*

b Aortic occlusion; collaterals:
- *Arise from visceral arteries,*
- *Pass to IIA branches.*

Reproduced from Fig. 12.16a,b, from Myers KA, Marshall RD, Freidin J. Principles of Pathology. Oxford: Blackwell, 1980 with permission from Blackwell.

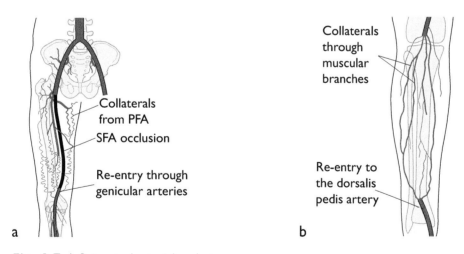

Fig. 6.7 *Infrainguinal arterial occlusions.*
a SFA occlusion; collaterals:
- *Arise from PFA and SFA branches,*
- *Pass to genicular arteries at the knee.*

b Popliteal and infrapopliteal artery occlusion; collaterals:
- *Arise from genicular arteries,*
- *Pass through muscular branches to reform distal infrapopliteal arteries.*

Reproduced from Figs 12.16d and 12.17b, Myers KA, Marshall RD, Freidin J. Principles of Pathology. Oxford: Blackwell, 1980 with permission from Blackwell.

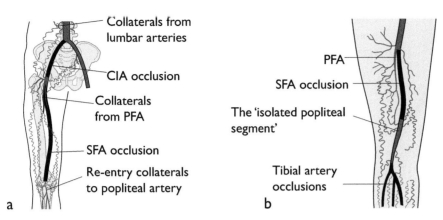

Fig. 6.8 *Multiple arterial occlusions.*
a *CIA and SFA occlusions; collaterals:*
  • *Arise from parietal and visceral arteries and IIA branches,*
  • *Re-enter the isolated CFA segment,*
  • *Pass from PFA branches through genicular arteries to the popliteal artery.*
b *SFA and infrapopliteal artery occlusions; collaterals:*
  • *Arise from branches of the PFA,*
  • *Re-enter the isolated popliteal segment,*
  • *Pass from genicular arteries to muscular branches to the leg.*

Reproduced from Figs 12.16i and 12.17a, Myers KA, Marshall RD, Freidin J. Principles of Pathology. Oxford: Blackwell, 1980 with permission from Blackwell.

Frequency for predominant disease at each level
● Aortoiliac ≈ 25%
● Femoropopliteal ≈ 65%
● Infrapopliteal ≈ 10%, more frequent in people with diabetes.

Clinical presentations
● The severity of symptoms (Fig. 6.9) depends on several factors:
  ○ Which arteries are involved,
  ○ The extent and number of lesions,
  ○ Whether there is stenosis or occlusion,
  ○ The extent of collaterals.

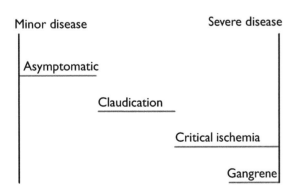

Fig. 6.9 *The range of clinical presentations.*
Reproduced from Fig. 8.3, Myers KA, Sumner DS, Nicolaides AN. Lower Limb Ischaemia. London: Medorion, 1997.

- Clinical examination is directed towards the following features:
  - The appearance of the legs and feet.
  - Palpation of the femoral, popliteal, posterior tibial and dorsalis pedis pulses to determine if they are normal, reduced or absent.
  - Use of a stethoscope to detect bruits over the upper and mid-abdomen, inguinal region, adductor hiatus and popliteal fossa, at rest and after exercise.

Intermittent claudication

- Characteristic features of intermittent claudication (*claudicare* – to limp):
  - Reproducible muscle pain with exercise,
  - Alternately, fatigue, heaviness, or tightness with exercise,
  - Walking distance reduced on an incline,
  - Distance to claudication constant,
  - Relief after rest for 3–5 min.
- Sites of claudication:
  - It may be limited to the calf with disease at any level.
  - Pain in the thigh as well as calf always indicates disease proximal to the SFA.
  - Buttock claudication indicates disease in the aorta, CIAs or IIAs.
  - Occasionally claudication is isolated to the buttock with IIA disease, the thigh with PFA disease or the foot with infrapopliteal artery disease.

Critical ischemia

- More severe ischemia is commonly due to disease at multiple levels.
- Rest pain occurs particularly at night.
- Ischemic ulceration can develop over pressure points or sites of trauma.
- Gangrene (infarction with secondary putrefaction) usually affects toes but can occur on the heel or anterior tibial compartment.
- Multiple small emboli can cause 'blue toe syndrome'.

Leriche's syndrome*

- Occlusion of the abdominal aorta can cause three features:
  - Buttock, thigh and calf claudication.
  - Impotence.
  - Diminished or absent femoral pulses.

Differential diagnosis

- Consider the following alternate diagnoses if leg pain is not clearly associated with exercise, but occurs with standing, sitting, or lying down, or is not alleviated by rest:
  - Sciatica or other neurogenic causes.
  - Spinal canal stenosis.
  - Arthritis.
  - Musculoskeletal causes.
  - Venous claudication.

---

*René Leriche, 1879–1955, French surgeon

Treatment

- Various options relate to the severity of the disease (Fig. 6.10).
- Disease commonly involves more than one segment and it can be difficult to assess the relative contribution from each.
- Symptoms are not relieved if the incorrect segment is treated.

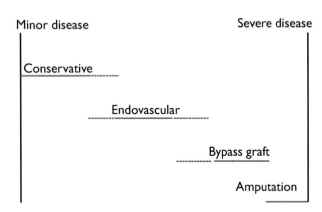

Minor disease   Severe disease

Conservative

Endovascular

Bypass graft

Amputation

Fig. 6.10 *Varying indications for each treatment option shown by overlap of the lines.*

Reproduced from Fig. 8.4, Myers, KA, Sumner DS, Nicolaides AN. Lower Limb Ischaemia. London: Medorion, 1997.

Conservative management

- Most patients with intermittent claudication should continue walking in spite of pain and modify risk factors for atherosclerosis.
- Improvement is at least as likely as deterioration so that intervention may never be required.

Endovascular intervention

- Many stenoses or occlusions can be effectively treated by balloon dilatation or stenting (Fig. 6.11).

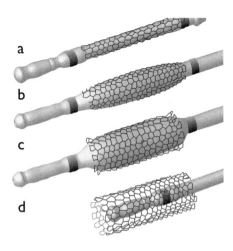

a

b

c

d

Fig. 6.11 *A balloon-expandable stent:*
a *Balloon deflated and stent collapsed,*
b *Balloon inflating,*
c *Balloon fully inflated,*
d *Stent fully expanded and balloon withdrawn.*

Surgical endarterectomy

- The atherosclerosis and inner layers of the media are peeled out and the arterial incision is commonly patched with vein or synthetic material to widen the artery (Fig. 6.12).

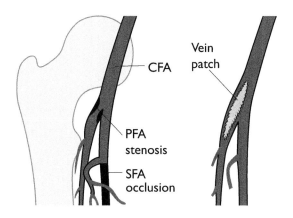

Fig. 6.12 *Profunda endarterectomy and patch.*

Reproduced from Fig. 12.18, Myers KA, Marshall RD, Freidin J. Principles of Pathology. Oxford: Blackwell, 1980 with permission from Blackwell.

Surgical bypass grafts

Autogenous vein

- A vein is preferred for infrainguinal bypass grafting (Fig. 6.13).
- The vein can be reversed so that valves do not impede flow or non-reversed *in situ* after breaking down valves and ligating tributaries.
- The ipsilateral or contralateral great or small saphenous veins or the arm veins can be used.
- These need to be scanned before surgery to ensure that they are large enough and not thrombosed.

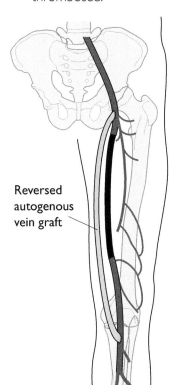

Fig. 6.13 *Reversed autogenous femoropopliteal vein bypass graft.*

Reproduced from Fig. 5.9, Myers KA, Marshall RD, Freidin J. Principles of Pathology. Oxford: Blackwell, 1980 with permission from Blackwell.

Synthetic grafts
● Grafts made from Dacron or polytetrafluoroethylene (PTFE) are used for intra-abdominal arterial disease (Fig. 6.14).
● They may be used for infrainguinal grafts with an above-knee distal anastomosis or when suitable vein cannot be found.
● Composite grafts combining autogenous vein and a synthetic material can be used.

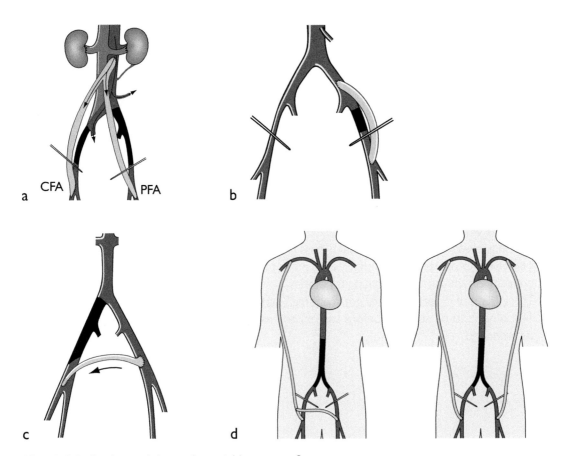

Fig. 6.14 *Synthetic abdominal arterial bypass grafts:*
a *Aortobifemoral bypass.*
b *Iliofemoral bypass.*
c *Femorofemoral bypass.*
d *Unilateral or bilateral axillofemoral bypass.*

(a) is reproduced from Fig. 13.10, Queral L. In: Bergan JJ, Yao JS. Surgery of the Aorta and its Body Branches. New York: Grune & Stratton 1979 with permission.

Amputation
● Major below-knee or above-knee amputation may be required in patients with critical ischemia where there is no runoff artery to accept the distal anastomosis for a bypass graft.

CLINICAL ASPECTS – ANEURYSMS

Regional pathology

- The distribution of aneurysms is different to that for occlusive disease (Fig. 6.15).
- Ultrasound surveillance shows that an abdominal aortic aneurysm (AAA) expands on average by 3–4 mm/year.
- An AAA is unlikely to rupture until it reaches 5–5.5 cm in diameter and the corresponding diameter for iliac aneurysms is approximately 3 cm.
- As an AAA expands, laminated thrombus may accumulate on the aortic wall to maintain a normal flow channel.
- Approximately 30% of patients with AAAs also have popliteal aneurysms and vice versa.

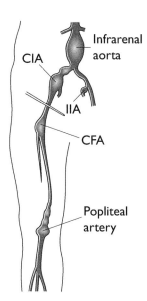

Fig. 6.15 *Common sites for aneurysms in arteries to the lower limbs.*
- *The infrarenal abdominal aorta, CIA, CFA or popliteal artery.*

Reproduced from Fig. 12.19, Myers KA, Marshall RD, Freidin J. Principles of Pathology. Oxford: Blackwell, 1980 with permission from Blackwell.

Clinical presentations

Abdominal aortic aneurysms

- Asymptomatic AAAs are usually diagnosed by chance and there are several presentations:
    - A pulsatile abdominal mass noticed by the patient.
    - Clinical palpation, although many large AAAs are not detected in obese patients, whereas a tortuous aorta can be misdiagnosed as an AAA in a thin patient.
    - Detection by a plain radiograph showing calcification in the wall.
    - Ultrasound or CT for other abdominal or pelvic pathology.
- Embolism of mural thrombus can cause '*blue-toe syndrome*'.
- Retroperitoneal leakage or rupture will cause sudden severe abdominal or low back pain or shock.

CFA aneurysm

- Palpable mass in the groin.
- Rupture.
- Distal ischemia from thrombosis.

Popliteal aneurysm
- Palpable popliteal fossa mass.
- Distal ischemia from thrombosis.
- Calf muscle dysfunction and numbness from posterior tibial nerve compression.
- Calf swelling due to venous compression.

Treatment
AAA
- AAAs can be treated by open aortic bypass grafting (Fig. 6.16).
- Many AAAs are now treated by endovascular aneurysm repair (EVAR), inserting a self-expanding endoluminal stent-graft through the CFAs inside the AAA with stents anchoring the proximal and distal ends (Fig. 6.17).

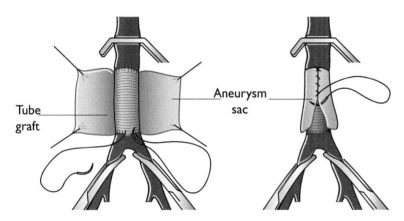

Fig. 6.16 *Tube graft for AAA.*
- *A Dacron tube is anastomosed end to end to the infrarenal aorta and aortic bifurcation. The aneurysm sac is closed around the graft to separate it from overlying bowel.*

Reproduced from Fig. 13.10 in: Bergan JJ, Yao JS. Surgery of the Aorta and its Body Branches. New York: Grune & Stratton, 1979 with permission.

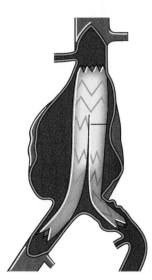

Fig. 6.17 *Endovascular aneurysm repair.*
- *The stent-graft expands to make firm circumferential contact with a 'neck' of relatively normal aorta between the renal arteries and the upper end of the AAA, as well as each CIA below the aneurysm.*

- Fenestrated stent-grafts are used if it is necessary to place the proximal end above renal, superior mesenteric arteries or the celiac axis due to proximal aneurysm extension. They are constructed with gaps positioned opposite one or more of each arterial branch orifice so that one or more further covered straight stent-grafts can be passed through each opening to preserve their circulation.
- EVAR is possible only if there is a proximal neck and distal site for anchoring each end of the stent-graft. Fenestrated stent-grafts now make this possible in most patients.

CFA and popliteal artery aneurysms
- These are treated by synthetic or vein grafts or endovascular stent-grafts.

Endoleaks after EVAR (Fig. 6.18)
- This complication where blood leaks into the original AAA is classified as follows:
  - *Type I*: loss of contact between either end of graft and artery:
    - Leak at proximal end of graft.
    - Leak at distal end of graft.
  - *Type II*: flow into the sac from reversed flow in the inferior mesenteric or lumbar arteries or other aortic branches.
  - *Type III*: flow through a tear in the fabric of the graft or between modular components.
  - *Type IV*: flow through interstices of the graft material.
  - *Type V*: sac expansion with no demonstrated leak.

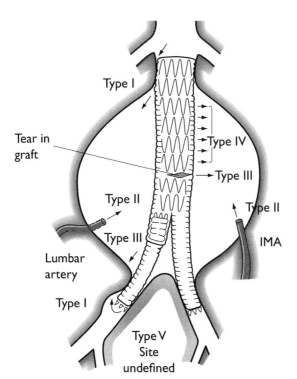

Fig. 6.18 *Types of endoleaks after an EVAR repair.*

CLINICAL ASPECTS – NON-ATHEROSCLEROTIC DISEASES

- Pathology for several conditions is discussed more extensively in Chapter 2.
- Other diseases are specific for arteries to the lower extremity.
- All of the conditions described below have characteristic ultrasound features, but all apart from tibial compartment syndrome are better evaluated by digital subtraction angiography (DSA), computed tomography angiography (CTA) or magnetic resonance angiography (MRA).

Regional pathology, presentation, and treatment
Popliteal entrapment syndrome (Fig. 6.19)

- This results from an abnormal course of the popliteal artery in relation to the medial head of gastrocnemius or other muscles.
- Repeated trauma may lead to stenosis, post-stenotic aneurysm or thrombosis.
- Duplex scanning can show some degree of popliteal artery and vein compression in normal individuals, particularly trained athletes with large muscles.
- It is classified into five types:
  - ○ *Type I:* the artery is displaced medial to the muscle origin (60–75% of patients).
  - ○ *Type II:* the artery descends in a straight course medial to the muscle which arises more lateral than normal.
  - ○ *Type III:* the artery descends in a straight course medial to an accessory slip of muscle.
  - ○ *Type IV:* the artery is trapped by popliteus, soleus, or plantaris, or a fibrous band.
  - ○ *Type V:* there is no obvious anatomical abnormality.
- Presentation is with intermittent claudication, particularly running backwards or walking up stairs.
- Treatment is by surgical division of the structure causing entrapment.

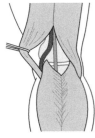
Type I

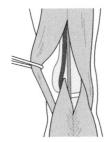
Type II

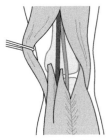
Type III

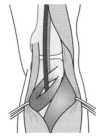
Type IV

Fig. 6.19 *Popliteal artery entrapment.*
Reproduced from Fig. 25.5, Myers, KA, Sumner DS, Nicolaides AN. Lower Limb Ischaemia. London: Medorion, 1997.

Abdominal aortic coarctation
- A congenital aortic stricture can cause renovascular and lower limb ischemia.
- Treatment is by surgical bypass grafting.

Aortic dissection
- A thoracic aortic dissection commonly extends into the abdominal aorta.
- Abdominal aortic dissection alone is rare.
- This is usually a complication of hypertension.
- Distal extension of dissection can occlude one or both common iliac arteries.
- Presentation is with acute severe lower limb ischemia.
- Treatment is by endovascular stent-grafting.

Takayasu's ('pulseless') disease
- This is intimal fibrosis that may cause stenoses in the aorta and large branches of the aorta.
- The disease can cause occlusion of multiple visceral branches.
- An aortic aneurysm may develop.
- Presentation is with intermittent claudication or critical ischemia.
- There are specific features for ultrasound but the condition is best evaluated by CTA and DSA.
- Treatment is by surgical bypass grafting.

Buerger's disease
- The condition characteristically affects infrapopliteal arteries.
- It causes multiple occlusions and copious collaterals.
- There is usually little or no involvement of arteries above the knees.
- It affects young males who are smokers.
- Presentation is frequently with critical ischemia leading to distal gangrene.
- Treatment is by surgical bypass grafting if possible.
- Many patients go on to amputation, particularly if they continue smoking.

Giant cell arteritis
- This is inflammatory thickening of the aortic wall.
- An inflammatory aortic aneurysm may develop.
- Medical treatment is preferred but surgical bypass grafting may be required for an aortic aneurysm.

Fibromuscular dysplasia
- This occasionally affects external iliac arteries.
- There may or may not be associated renal artery involvement.
- As with the condition at other sites, it is most frequent in young females.
- Presentation is with intermittent claudication.
- Treatment may require surgical bypass grafting.

Post-irradiation arteritis
- This complication usually follows irradiation for pelvic tumors such as carcinoma of the uterus.
- It can cause common or external iliac stenosis or occlusion.
- Presentation is with intermittent claudication.
- Treatment is by surgical bypass grafting from arteries well away from the irradiated region.

Ergotism

- This causes diffuse spasm or late occlusion of larger iliac and femoral arteries rather than their smaller branches.
- Presentation is with intermittent claudication of short duration.
- Most symptoms resolve after stopping the ergot derivative drug treatment.

Repetitive external iliac arterial trauma

- Tethering of the iliac artery by the psoas arterial branch and fibrous tissue predisposes the artery to kinking and compression, e.g. during cycling.
- This causes subintimal fibrosis.
- Characteristic findings are long stenoses from just beyond the EIA origin with lengthening and tortuosity of the artery.
- Presentation is with intermittent claudication.
- Treatment involves surgical patch grafting.

Cystic adventitial disease

- This can affect the popliteal artery or vein and causes popliteal artery stenosis which can progress to a short occlusion.
- Gelatinous material accumulates in the adventitia to cause smooth narrowing of the lumen with normal proximal and distal arteries.
- The condition is usually seen in young males.
- The diagnosis is confirmed by DSA.
- Presentation is with intermittent claudication.
- Treatment is by surgical patch or bypass grafting.

Tibial compartment syndrome

- The condition most often affects the anterior compartment.
- It commences with impaired venous outflow, leading to increased compartmental pressure and restricted arterial inflow.
- Clinical manifestations can range from aching to ischemic necrosis.
- The diagnosis is confirmed by pressure studies in the affected tibial compartments.
- Treatment is by fasciotomy.

Persistent sciatic artery (PSA) (Fig. 6.20)

- PSA arises from the IIA and passes through the greater sciatic notch down the back of the thigh.
- It joins a normal popliteal artery in 90%, but an incomplete form terminates at the back of the thigh in 10%.
- The SFA is normal in 15% but hypoplastic or absent in the remainder.
- Either the PSA or the SFA provides a normal circulation in >95%, and <5% have incomplete arteries and ischemia.
- PSA is bilateral in 25%.
- About 50% have an aneurysm just distal to the sciatic notch, particularly if the SFA is hypoplastic or absent.
- Presentation is with intermittent claudication at a young age if the circulation is incomplete.
- Treatment is by surgical bypass grafting if the circulation is incomplete.
- Endovascular stent-grafting may be required for an iliac aneurysm.

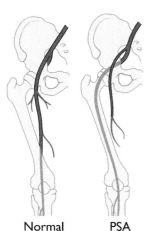

Normal   PSA

Fig. 6.20 *Anatomy of persistent sciatic artery.*

WHAT DOCTORS NEED TO KNOW

Atherosclerotic occlusive disease
- What are the sites of disease?
- Are there multiple segments?
- Is each a stenosis or occlusion?
- What is the severity of stenosis?
- What is the length of each lesion?
- What is the location of the lesion?

AAA and iliac aneurysms
- What is the maximum diameter and length?
- Is there mural thrombus and what is the residual lumen diameter?
- What is the length of normal aorta between the lowest renal artery and the upper end of the AAA?
- Where does the AAA finish in relation to the aortic bifurcation or iliac arteries?
- Is the aortic bifurcation involved?
- What are the maximum diameters of iliac aneurysms and the unaffected iliac arteries?
- Where are iliac aneurysms located and what are their lengths?
- What are the diameters of the CFAs?

Infrainguinal aneurysm
- What is the position and extent?
- What are its dimensions?
- Is there mural thrombus and what is the residual lumen diameter?
- Is it patent or occluded?

Non-atherosclerotic disease
- What is the disease or syndrome?
- Which arteries are affected?
- What is its severity?
- What is its extent?

THE DUPLEX SCAN

- An experienced sonographer can scan arteries from the aorta to feet in both limbs in a reasonable time in >90% of well-prepared patients.
- Ultrasound can detect major artery disease with >90% accuracy when compared with DSA.
- Distal disease may be less accurately assessed by ultrasound if there are multiple stenoses.

Abbreviations

- Peak systolic velocity (cm/s) – PSV
- End-diastolic velocity (cm/s) – EDV
- Ratio of PSV at and just proximal to a stenosis – PSV ratio – V_2/V_1
- Pansystolic spectral broadening – PSB.

OPINION!

- **A good history and clinical examination are sufficient to assess many patients with typical symptoms and mild disability, without the need to involve the vascular diagnostic service.**

Indications for scanning

Occlusive arterial disease

- Patients with equivocal symptoms or obscure diagnosis.
- Patients with clinical symptoms sufficient to warrant intervention using ultrasound to:
  - Locate sites of serious disease to precisely plan for arteriography.
  - Select patients for endovascular therapy without prior arteriography.
- If the ultrasound scan is equivocal then this warrants a diagnostic arteriogram to:
  - Distinguish tight stenosis from occlusion.
  - Assess contribution from multiple stenoses.
  - Detect and grade disease in infrapopliteal arteries.

Monitoring at completion of infrainguinal bypass grafting

- Some surgeons scan the arterial bypass graft in the operating theatre before completing the procedure.
- Raised velocities, kinking, twist or thrombus indicate the need for revision to prevent early occlusion.
- Low flow suggests the need for a distal arteriovenous fistula or sequential distal bypass graft to augment flow.
- Any abnormality may be an indication for aggressive postoperative antithrombotic treatment.

Surveillance after infrainguinal bypass grafting

- Bypass grafts are subject to stenosis or occlusion (Fig. 6.21):
  - First few weeks – technical faults.
  - First 2 years – neointimal hyperplasia in the graft and at the anastomoses.
  - After 2 years – atherosclerosis in the graft and inflow and outflow arteries.
  - Long term – graft degeneration.
- Graft stenosis may not cause recurrent symptoms and can be detected by ultrasound surveillance although some grafts occlude without prior stenosis.
- There is strong support for surveillance after autogenous vein grafting. The graft is monitored for the following:
  - Increased or reduced PSV in the graft, and inflow and outflow arteries.
  - Occlusion.
  - Incorporation into surrounding tissues.
- Traditional intervals for graft surveillance:
  - 1 month after operation.
  - 3-monthly for 1 year.
  - Biannually for the second year.
  - Annually thereafter.
- There is less support for routine surveillance after a synthetic graft or endovascular procedure than for a vein bypass graft but a positive finding can lead to correction of restenosis.

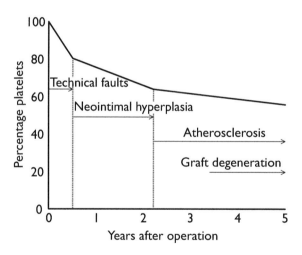

Fig. 6.21 Causes of graft failure.
Redrawn from Fig. 11.1, van Reedt Dortland RWH. In: Chant ADB, Barros D'Sa AAB (eds), Emergency Vascular Practice. London: Hodder Arnold, 1997 with permission.

Detection of AAA and iliac aneurysms

- Screening programs have been introduced in many countries to offer ultrasound assessment to detect AAA and iliac aneurysms.
- They are particularly targeted at older males, individuals with a family history of AAA and individuals with risk factors for AAA.

Surveillance for AAA and iliac aneurysms

- If no intervention is performed, annual reviews are required to determine any increase in size to the stage at which risk of rupture becomes high:
  - AAA – diameter ≥ 5 cm.
  - Iliac aneurysm – diameter ≥3 cm.
- Vascular ultrasound is a simple and reliable technique to assess an AAA if intervention is being considered (Fig. 6.22) although other investigations are also required before intervention.

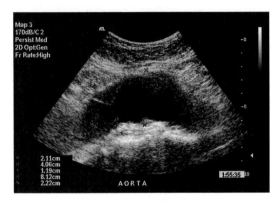

Fig. 6.22 *B-mode of an AAA.*
- *Longitudinal view showing diameter of the neck, maximum anteroposterior diameter, residual lumen diameter, aneurysm length, and distal aortic diameter.*

Surveillance after EVAR for AAA

- Surveillance is required after EVAR.
- Primary surveillance ultrasound for a fenestrated stent-graft should not be undertaken before 48–72 hours post-insertion.
- The most important complication is endoleak from within the graft back into the AAA sac, and this is well seen with duplex scanning (Fig. 6.23).
- The scan for a fenestrated stent-graft includes examining the renal arteries, superior mesenteric artery and celiac axis orifices for stent stenoses.
- Type II endoleaks mostly resolve on their own accord.
- Type III endoleaks need prompt repair.
- Type IV endoleaks are now rarely seen.
- Alternating ultrasound and CT reduces radiation exposure and limits contrast dye in patients with chronic renal insufficiency.
- Integrity and a stable position are best shown by serial plain radiographs.

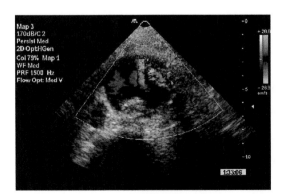

Fig. 6.23 *Color Doppler image of a Type I endoleak from an endoluminal graft.*

Normal findings

- A high-resistance bi- or triphasic signal with no PSB.
- PSV no higher than 150 cm/s (*Table 6.1*).

Table 6.1 *Representative normal peak systolic velocities (PSVs) in lower limb arteries.*

Artery	PSV (cm/s)
Aorta	75
CIA	110
EIA	110
CFA	90
Proximal SFA	90
Distal SFA	75
Popliteal	60
Infrapopliteal	50

Criteria for diagnosing occlusive disease
Lower limb arterial stenoses

- These have been defined by comparing the maximum PSV or PSV ratio and waveform analysis with DSA.
- We use criteria derived by Cossman and colleagues* (*Table 6.2*).
- There is no consensus as to whether the PSV or PSV ratio is more accurate although the PSV ratio may be preferred for multiple stenoses.
- With increasing degrees of stenosis, the waveform shows progressive PSB and then post-stenotic turbulence.

Table 6.2 *Criteria for diagnosing lower limb arterial stenoses.*

Stenosis (%)	PSV (cm/s)	V_2/V_1 ratio
30–50	150–200	1.5–2
50–75	200–400	2–4
>75	>400	>4
>90	–	>7

*Cossman D, Ellison JE, Wagner WH, *et al.* Comparison of contrast arteriography to arterial mapping with color-flow duplex imaging in the lower extremities. *J Vasc Surg* 1989; **10**:522–9

- Severe stenosis may be associated with aliasing, monophasic or forward and reverse flow, and a shrill high-velocity signal.
- An image for spectral analysis of a >75% stenosis of an SFA is shown in Fig. 6.24.

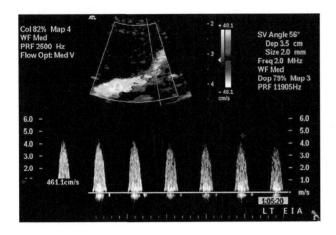

Fig. 6.24 *Spectral analysis for SFA >75% stenosis.*

Plaque characteristics
- Composition and echogenicity:
  - Homogeneous
  - Heterogeneous
  - Calcified
  - Cauliflower calcified
  - Echogenic
  - Echolucent.
- Surface:
  - Smooth
  - Irregular.

Intraoperative monitoring for infrainguinal bypass graft
- PSV >180 cm/s, spectral broadening, PSV ratio >3.0, kinking, twist or thrombus indicates a fault in the graft.
- PSV <30–40 cm/s and absent diastolic flow suggest inadequate flow to maintain patency.

Infrainguinal bypass graft stenosis
- Most departments use a PSV ratio to define significant graft stenosis with discriminant values reported from >1.5 to >3.0.
- A maximum PSV >350 cm/s or <45 cm/s also suggests imminent graft failure.
- Changes in the spectral waveform from tri- or biphasic to monophasic in the graft or inflow arteries indirectly predict graft stenosis.

Lower limb arterial occlusion
- Occlusion is diagnosed with confidence if the following are observed:
  - No color Doppler or spectral signal in the occluded segment,
  - High-resistance spectral signal above the segment,
  - Low-amplitude spectral signal below the segment,
  - A collateral leaving the artery at the proximal end,
  - A collateral re-entering the artery at the distal end.

AAA and other aneurysms

- An AAA is defined as a diameter >3 cm or a diameter increased by more than 1.5 times the proximal diameter.
- All other aneurysms are defined as a diameter increased by more than 1.5 times the proximal diameter.

Surveillance after EVAR

- The purpose is to detect an endoleak and classify its type, to measure change in the residual sac diameter and also to detect stenosis in major branches after fenestrated stent-grafts.
- An endoleak is probably present if the residual lumen diameter increases with surveillance and is not present if the AAA residual diameter has decreased.
- Type I endoleak is present if color, spectral and power Doppler show flow from the top or bottom end of the graft into the residual sac.
- Type II endoleak is indicated by reverse flow on color and spectral Doppler in an aortic branch with color or power Doppler filling of the residual sac.
- Type III and IV endoleaks are indicated by color or power Doppler flow escaping into the residual sac from the body of the graft.
- Type V endoleak is demonstrated by an increase in sac diameter with no demonstration of leak on color or power Doppler.
- Indirect evidence of endoleak:
  - EVAR migration.
  - Increase in sac size.
  - Increased sac pulsatility.
- Surveillance may be discontinued if the sac disappears.

Popliteal entrapment syndrome

- This is diagnosed by finding a normal PSV at rest with an increased PSV to ≥ 200 cm/s or flow cessation with isometric active ankle plantarflexion or passive forced ankle dorsiflexion (Fig. 6.25).
- The popliteal artery is either partially or fully compressed in provocative positions.
- Dampened flow in distal infrapopliteal arteries when in provocative positions may aid diagnosis.

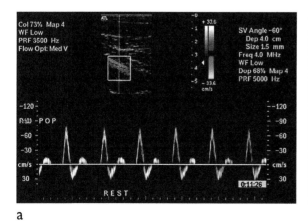 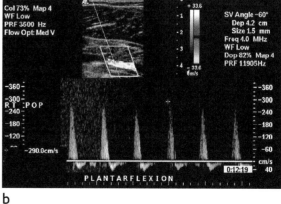

a   b

Fig. 6.25 *Spectral Doppler signals in a popliteal artery with popliteal entrapment syndrome:*
a *At rest.*
b *During active isometric plantarflexion.*

Abdominal aortic coarctation

- B-mode and color Doppler evidence of aortic constriction.
- Spectral Doppler evidence of stenosis at the level of constriction.

Aortic dissection

- Visualization of an intimal flap.
- Ultrasound may show a long narrow residual lumen.
- On color Doppler there may be multiple sites of entry and exit of flow.
- There may be ultrasound evidence of iliac dissection.

Takayasu's ('pulseless') disease

- A characteristic ultrasound feature is homogeneous circumferential intima–media thickening of the aorta.
- There is ultrasound evidence of occlusion or stenosis of the aorta with possible involvement of large aortic branches.
- AAAs may also be observed on ultrasound.

Buerger's disease

- There is color and spectral Doppler evidence of occlusions with collateral flow in the infrapopliteal and occasionally popliteal arteries.

Giant cell arteritis

- Characteristic appearances are circumferential hypoechogenic homogeneous thickening of the aortic wall.
- A 'halo' appearance around the aorta is seen on ultrasound.

Fibromuscular dysplasia

- 'String-of-beads' appearance on ultrasound.
- Associated stenoses present.

Post-irradation arteritis

- Circumferential hypoechogenic homogeneous thickening of the common or external iliac arteries.
- Color and spectral Doppler may demonstrate associated stenosis or occlusion.

Ergotism

- Ultrasound demonstration of arterial spasm.
- Color and spectral Doppler can indicate associated occlusion.

Repetitive external iliac arterial trauma

- Color and spectral Doppler evidence of a long stenosis from just beyond the origin of the EIA.
- Lengthening and tortuosity of the EIA with B-mode evidence of fibrosis.

Cystic adventitial disease

- Evidence of the 'scimitar sign' showing single or multiple anechoic to hypoechoic cysts displacing the popliteal artery to one side.
- No color flow demonstrated in the lesions.
- There may be spectral evidence of associated stenosis.

Tibial compartment syndrome
- B-mode and color Doppler demonstrate constriction of the anterior tibial vein and possibly the artery.
- Spectral Doppler demonstrates reduced flow.

Persistent sciatic artery
- Ultrasound evidence of hypoplastic or absent SFA.
- Patent PSA in the posterior thigh.

PROTOCOLS FOR SCANNING
- Preparing the patient, selecting the best transducer and general principles for scanning are discussed in Chapter 3 (pages 35–37).

OPINION!
- **We consider that aortoiliac arteries should be scanned as part of the initial study for any patient being investigated for lower limb arterial disease.**
- **We do not consider that it is sufficient to infer whether aortoiliac disease is present or absent from indirect assessment of CFA waveforms.**

Aorta
Position the patient and select windows
- Scan with the patient lying in supine position.
- Image from an anterior approach through rectus abdominis to the left of the midline, superior to the umbilicus and at the umbilical level.
- Turn the patient to right lateral decubitus position and use a coronal (flank) window if the patient is gassy or obese.
- Tilt the table at various angles to shift gas to different positions in the bowel.
- Use the transducer to massage the abdomen from lateral to medial to manipulate bowel gas.

Scan for occlusive disease
- In B-mode and transverse, measure the maximum infrarenal diameter.
- Use B-mode to classify plaque type.
- Use color Doppler in longitudinal to highlight aliasing. Walk the spectral Doppler sample through areas of color aliasing.
- Use spectral Doppler to obtain PSVs proximal to, at and distal to stenosis to classify severity, location, and extent.
- Describe location of stenosis as suprarenal, proximal, mid or distal infrarenal aorta.

Scan for aneurysmal disease

- Measure the true maximum transverse diameter in B-mode (Fig. 6.26), then change to longitudinal to measure the maximum anteroposterior diameter.
- In B-mode, note mural thrombus and record the minimum residual lumen diameter.
- Use color Doppler to help show the lumen if mural thrombus is echolucent.
- In B-mode, measure diameters proximal and distal to the AAA.
- Note if dilation extends suprarenally, if it involves the renal arteries or aortic bifurcation and if tortuosity is present.
- Record the relation of the upper end of the AAA to the renal arteries and measure the length of neck from the most inferior renal artery.

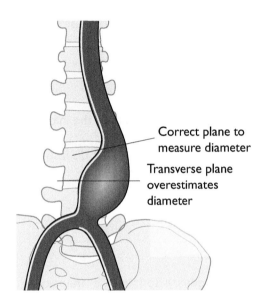

Correct plane to measure diameter

Transverse plane overestimates diameter

Fig. 6.26 *Transverse diameter of an AAA.*
- *Measure the true oblique diameter rather than the transverse plane, which will overestimate the diameter if the aorta and AAA are tortuous.*

Scan for surveillance after EVAR

- Reduce color scale to highlight low-velocity flow.
- Increase color persistence.
- Use spectral Doppler to demonstrate flow direction in branches of the aorta.
- Use B-mode to measure diameters of the residual lumen of the AAA and limbs of the graft.
- With color Doppler, scan throughout the residual sac looking for flow and identify the origin of flow to classify endoleak type.
- With color Doppler, examine for intermittent endoleak with the patient supine and in right and left lateral decubitus.
- For a fenestrated graft, obtain sample spectral traces within the stented orifices of aortic branches to identify the presence of stenosis.

Iliac arteries
Position the patient and select windows

- Scan with the patient lying supine.
- Image from an oblique approach to separate the iliac arteries and veins.
- Lateral decubitus positions with coronal (flank) windows are helpful if the patient is gassy or obese.

Scan the CIA, IIA, and EIA

- Some start at the aortic bifurcation and scan distally.
- Others start from the inguinal ligament and scan proximally.
- Identify and scan the iliac arteries in longitudinal with color Doppler.
- Use color Doppler in longitudinal to highlight aliasing. Walk the spectral Doppler sample through areas of color aliasing.
- Use color Doppler to identify the distal EIA curving towards the transducer and follow it proximally to the iliac bifurcation.
- Use color Doppler to identify the IIA passing deep into the pelvis.
- Continue to scan the CIA to the abdominal aorta which is recognized by a sudden increase in diameter at the umbilicus.
- Use B-mode to classify plaque type.
- Note if the iliac arteries are tortuous or ectatic; if so in B-mode measure maximum and minimum diameters.
- Take sample spectral traces and record PSVs proximal to, at and distal to sites of stenosis to assess severity, location, and extent.
- Describe stenosis location as origin, proximal, mid, distal or throughout.
- Take sample spectral traces proximal to, within and distal to occlusions to demonstrate extent and location from an anatomical landmark.
- If scanning an EVAR, examine the iliac residual sacs for endoleak and throughout the limb grafts and iliac arteries for stenosis or other complications.

NOTE!

- **Plaque and diameters must be classified with color turned off because this will increase spatial resolution.**

Groin and thigh arteries

Position the patient and select windows

- Scan with the patient lying supine and the limb externally rotated.
- Turn the patient if necessary.
- View the CFA and femoral bifurcation through the femoral triangle.
- Follow the SFA through an anteromedial aspect.
- Image quality may deteriorate as the SFA passes through the hiatus in adductor magnus in the lower third of the thigh.
- Try straightening the leg and use an anterior approach through vastus medialis – the artery is further from the transducer but the image is improved.

Scan the CFA, PFA and SFA

- Commence in longitudinal in the CFA just proximal to the inguinal ligament and progress down to the femoral bifurcation.
- Turn into transverse and use B-mode and color Doppler to help identify the SFA and PFA origins.
- The PFA is lateral and deep to the SFA but it can be difficult to differentiate the two if either is occluded. The PFA has multiple branches.

- The femoral bifurcation is the landmark for measuring the origin and length of a stenosis or occlusion in the SFA.
- Use color Doppler to follow arteries in longitudinal and to highlight aliasing. Walk the spectral Doppler sample through areas of color aliasing.
- Take sample spectral traces and record PSVs proximal to, at and distal to sites of stenosis to classify severity, location and extent.
- Take sample spectral traces proximal to, within and distal to occlusions to demonstrate extent and location from an anatomical landmark.
- If there is a CFA aneurysm, use B-mode to measure its maximum diameter (Fig. 6.27) and diameters in the normal artery just proximal and distal.

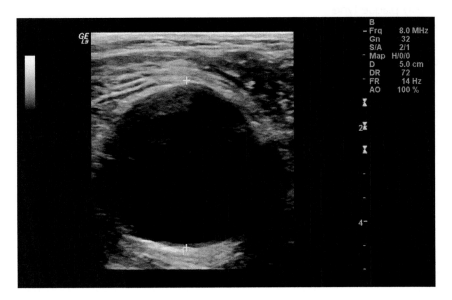

Fig. 6.27 *Transverse B-mode image of CFA aneurysm.*
- *Note the presence of mural thrombus.*

Image kindly supplied by Martin Necas, Hamilton, New Zealand.

TIP!

- **Use the adjacent vein as a guide if the SFA is occluded remembering that the vein is deep to the artery.**

Popliteal fossa arteries
Position the patient and select windows
- Turn the patient prone or in lateral decubitus with the knee slightly flexed to provide a posterior window.

Scan the popliteal artery and TPT
- Use B-mode and color Doppler in transverse to identify the popliteal artery.
- Turn the transducer to show the popliteal artery in longitudinal.

- Use color Doppler to determine arterial patency and indicate location of stenoses and occlusions. Walk the spectral Doppler sample through areas of color aliasing.
- Record sample spectral traces from at least one point in the popliteal artery.
- Record PSVs proximal to, at and distal to sites of stenosis, and classify the severity, extent and location from an anatomical landmark.
- Record spectral traces proximal to, within and distal to an occlusion to demonstrate extent and location from an anatomical landmark.
- Measure the position of stenosis or occlusion in relation to the skin crease at the back of the knee, or from the femoral bifurcation if a SFA stenosis is also present.
- If there is a popliteal aneurysm, use B-mode to measure its proximal, maximum and distal diameters.
- Note the presence of mural thrombus and record residual diameter.
- In longitudinal with color Doppler, scan throughout the TPT; use spectral Doppler to confirm patency if calcification from shadowing is making determination of patency difficult.
- Record a sample spectral trace in the TPT.

Scan for popliteal entrapment syndrome
- Use color Doppler in longitudinal to highlight areas of compression and associated aliasing. Walk the spectral Doppler sample through areas of color aliasing.
- Record sample spectral traces and measure PSVs in the distal popliteal artery, TPT and origin of the ATA with the foot at rest, in passive forced dorsiflexion, active plantarflexion and any provocative movement that induces symptoms.
- In B-mode, measure the diameter of the distal popliteal artery with the foot in the above-described positions.
- Always test both legs.

Infrapopliteal arteries
Position the patient and select windows
- Scan for the ATA through an anterolateral window with the patient supine and toes inverted.
- Scan for the PTA and peroneal artery from a medial approach with the patient supine and leg flexed to drop gastrocnemius away. Considerable transducer pressure may be required.
- An alternate method to view infrapopliteal arteries is to sit the patient with the foot on your knee to allow the calf muscles to drop away from the arteries and better fill veins as landmarks for the arteries.

Scan the ATA, PTA and peroneal artery
- Use B-mode and color Doppler in transverse to identify the arteries.
- Turn the transducer to show the arteries in longitudinal.
- Veins are duplicated and lie next to each artery. Compress the foot or calf muscles to augment venous flow and help identify adjacent arteries.
- Use color Doppler to follow each artery from the malleolus to its origin. Walk the spectral Doppler sample through areas of color aliasing.
- Reduce the color scale if necessary because flow is often low compared with more proximal arteries.
- If none of the infrapopliteal arteries is patent, scan dorsalis pedis and the medial plantar arteries for patency because these can be used in distal anastomoses for bypass grafts.
- Flow in infrapopliteal arteries can be difficult to see if there is severe inflow disease.

- Record PSVs proximal to, at and distal to sites of stenosis and classify the severity, location and extent.
- Record spectral traces proximal to, within and distal to an occlusion to demonstrate extent and location.
- Describe the position of disease as at the origin, in the proximal, mid or distal artery or throughout.
- Record sample spectral traces from each distal infrapopliteal artery.

Scan bypass grafts

- Find the proximal anastomosis using B-mode and color Doppler.
- Look for regions of inflow stenosis proximal to and at the proximal anastomosis. In B-mode, examine the proximal anastomosis for an aneurysm.
- If an aneurysm is present, use B-mode to measure maximum diameters, proximal native artery and proximal graft diameters.
- Use color Doppler in longitudinal to follow the graft to its distal anastomosis looking for regions of stenosis. Walk the spectral Doppler sample through areas of color aliasing.
- In B-mode and color Doppler, examine the bypass graft for neointimal hyperplasia (Fig. 6.28) and atherosclerosis.
- Take sample spectral traces from the proximal, mid and distal graft and record PSVs proximal to, at and distal to stenosis to classify severity, extent, and location in relation to the graft origin.
- Examine the distal anastomosis for aneurysm and stenosis.
- Examine distal outflow for stenosis and patency.
- Monitor the graft for incorporation into surrounding tissues or perigraft collection.

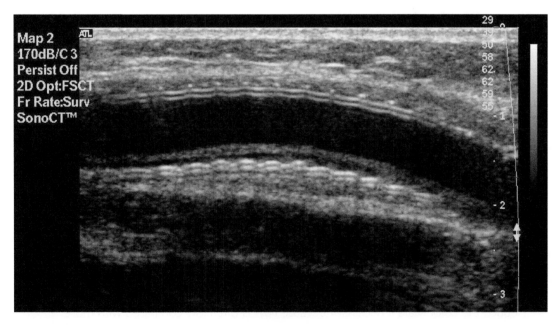

Fig. 6.28 *B-mode image of neointimal hyperplasia within a bypass graft.*
Image kindly supplied by Martin Necas, Hamilton, New Zealand.

TIPS!

- When scanning grafts, remember that they have no branches and usually lie superficial to the native artery and vein.
- The anastomosis sites are dilated in comparison to the native artery and graft.
- The serrated walls of a Dacron graft and the venous sinuses of an autogenous vein graft are easily identified.

OTHER INVESTIGATIONS

The ankle:brachial pressure index

- ABI = ankle systolic pressure/brachial systolic pressure.
- ABI helps to establish whether disease is present.

Technique

- Lay the patient supine.
- Rest the patient for a consistent baseline.
- Apply sphygmomanometer cuffs to each arm over the brachial artery.
- Locate the brachial artery with continuous-wave Doppler.
- Inflate the cuff to 20–30 mmHg above the last audible pulse and slowly deflate it.
- Record the systolic pressure when flow resumes – continuous wave is more accurate than the stethoscope in the arm.
- Apply cuffs at each ankle and follow the same procedure for each dorsalis pedis artery and PTA. The peroneal artery can be used if it is the only patent artery to the ankle. Note the anatomy from Fig. 6.4.
- Use the highest ankle pressure (dorsalis pedis or posterior tibial) and the highest of the two arm pressures to calculate the ABI.

WARNING!

- Cuffs should be applied snugly with the bladder over the artery to be compressed or otherwise spuriously high pressures will be recorded.

Other pressure indices

- Indices can also be calculated from thigh, calf, or toe pressures:
- Thigh pressures are normally recorded as higher than ankle or arm pressures (normal thigh:brachial index = 1.10–1.20). Wider cuffs are required.
- Toe pressures are measured by infrared photoplethysmography with a 1.2-cm-width cuff placed around the first toe. Toe pressures are normally recorded as lower than ankle or arm pressures (normal toe:brachial index = 0.80–0.90).

Treadmill studies

- The test measures walking distance and records systolic pressures at intervals after standard exercise on a treadmill.
- The walking distance measures disability and determines whether restriction agrees with the patient's history.

Technique

- Explain the procedure to the patient asking whether there are contraindications to exercise.
- Record resting ABIs. Leave the ankle cuffs on to allow for speedy assessment after exercise.
- Walk the patient on a motorized treadmill. A common protocol is to walk for up to 5 min at 2 km/h (33 m/min) on a 7° slope. If the patient cannot cope, reduce the speed and note the settings.
- ECG monitoring can be performed.
- Immediately after exercise, measure brachial and ankle pressures from the arteries that gave the highest readings before exercise and then obtain ankle pressures every minute until pressures return to normal or for no more than 10 min.
- Record the following:
  - Time for onset of leg pain.
  - Where it occurs.
  - Time when leg pain stops the patient from walking.
  - Resting and serial post-exercise ABIs until recovery to the pre-exercise pressure.
  - Any other reason for stopping:
    - Dyspnea.
    - Angina.
    - Joint pain.
    - Fatigue or debility.

WARNING!

- **Do not exercise a patient with daily exertional angina or myocardial infarct <3 months before unless medical staff are present.**
- **Avoid performing exercise tests if the brachial systolic pressure is >200 mmHg.**

Clinical applications

- If the resting ABI is reduced to <0.80 then occlusive disease is present. ABI >0.90 is considered normal.
- Differences in ABIs between the two limbs indicate whether disease is unilateral or bilateral and which is more severely affected if the disease is bilateral.
- If the resting ABI is normal but post-exercise ABIs fall then early occlusive disease is present. If the post-exercise ABI remains normal then symptomatic occlusive disease can usually be excluded.
- Exercise will cause a decrease in ABI relative to the resting value – any apparent rise is due to technical error.
- There is debate about the value of a post-exercise ABI if the resting ABI is already reduced.

- Observer variability is relatively high so that a decrease after exercise needs to be >0.15 to be significant.
- The test is invalid in some patients with heavily calcified infrapopliteal arteries that are incompressible, particularly in patients with diabetes.
- The ABI offers only an approximate estimate of disease severity.
- The ABI gives no information about where the disease is located.
- An increase in ABIs accurately reflects a satisfactory response to treatment by bypass surgery or balloon dilatation.
- A falling ABI predicts a failing graft.

WARNING!

- Do not inflate a cuff over a bypass graft or stent for fear of causing it to occlude.
- Inform the patient that cuff inflation can cause discomfort.

ULTRASOUND IMAGES TO RECORD

Atherosclerotic disease and graft surveillance
- Sample spectral traces in longitudinal for each artery listed.
- Spectral traces proximal to and at each stenosis; note the location from the anatomical landmark, the extent and the severity.
- Spectral traces proximal to, within and distal to occlusions; note the location from the anatomical landmark and extent.
- B-mode of plaques in longitudinal.
- Sample spectral traces in the artery above and below a bypass graft, anastomosis sites and proximal, mid and distal graft.
- B-mode diameters of any aneurysmal dilation at anastomosis sites and within the native artery and unaffected adjacent graft.
- B-mode image of any perigraft collections.

Aneurysms
- B-mode of length of aneurysm in longitudinal.
- B-mode of maximum transverse and anteroposterior diameters of aneurysm.
- B-mode of mural thrombus and residual lumen diameter of aneurysm.
- B-mode of proximal and distal diameters of adjacent normal artery.
- B-mode of distance of AAA from lowest renal artery.
- If AAA present, transverse B-mode diameters of iliac arteries and CFAs; note tortuosity.

EVAR surveillance
- Transverse B-mode images of maximum residual AAAs and iliac artery diameters.
- Transverse B-mode diameters of main, right and left graft limbs.
- Spectral traces demonstrating direction of flow in aortic branches.
- Color Doppler for endoleaks at all levels.

Popliteal entrapment syndrome
- Sample spectral traces in longitudinal for each artery listed.
- Sample spectral traces in the distal popliteal artery, TPT and origin of the ATA with the foot at rest, in passive forced dorsiflexion, active plantarflexion and any provocative movement that induces symptoms; note severity of transient stenosis.
- B-mode image of the diameter of the distal popliteal artery with the foot in the above-described positions.

Abdominal aortic coarctation
- Color image in longitudinal demonstrating aortic lumen constriction.
- B-mode measurements of diameters of maximum constriction, proximal and distal diameters of non-affected aorta.
- B-mode measurement of length of coarctation and location in relation to an abdominal aortic branch.
- Spectral traces proximal to and at maximum constriction; note severity of stenosis.

Aortic dissection
- B-mode and color images demonstrating a false lumen in the aorta in longitudinal and transverse.
- B-mode measurement of length of dissection and location in relation to an abdominal aorta branch.
- Sample spectral trace within false and true lumina.
- B-mode images and spectral traces from the iliac arteries.

Fibromuscular dysplasia
- Sample spectral traces in longitudinal for each artery listed.
- B-mode and color Doppler images in longitudinal demonstrating the 'string-of-beads' appearance in EIA.
- Spectral traces proximal to and at areas of stenoses; note the location, severity, and extent of stenoses.
- Spectral traces and color Doppler images of renal arteries.

Ergotism
- Sample spectral traces in longitudinal for each artery listed.
- Spectral traces demonstrating occlusions of iliac and femoral arteries; note the location from the anatomical landmark and the extent.
- Spectral traces in regions of spasm of iliac and femoral arteries.

Repetitive external iliac arterial trauma
- Sample spectral traces in longitudinal for each artery listed.
- B-mode images demonstrating wall thickening.
- Spectral traces proximal to, within, and distal to stenosis; note the location from the anatomical landmark, the extent, and the severity.
- Note areas of tortuosity in the EIA.

Buerger's disease
- Sample spectral traces in longitudinal for each artery listed.
- Spectral traces demonstrating occlusions below the knee; note the location from the anatomical landmark and the extent.

Giant cell arteritis, post-irradiation arteritis, and Takayasu's disease
- Sample spectral traces in longitudinal for each artery listed.
- B-mode longitudinal and transverse images demonstrating wall thickening and 'halo' appearance of affected artery.
- Spectral traces demonstrating occlusion or stenosis; note the location from anatomical landmarks, severity, and extent.

Cystic adventitial disease
- Sample spectral traces in longitudinal for each artery listed.
- B-mode and color images demonstrating the 'scimitar sign' in the popliteal artery.
- Spectral traces proximal to and at narrowing; note the location from the anatomical landmark, the extent and the severity.

Tibial compartment syndrome
- Sample spectral traces in longitudinal for each artery listed.
- B-mode and color images demonstrating constriction of the anterior tibial artery and vein.
- B-mode diameter measurements of constrictions.
- Spectral traces demonstrating reduced flow.
- Note location of constriction.

Persistent sciatic artery
- Sample spectral traces in longitudinal for each artery listed.
- B-mode and color images demonstrating hypoplastic or absent SFA.
- If SFA present, spectral traces to demonstrate reduced flow.
- Spectral traces to demonstrate that the PSA is the major inflow artery.

WORKSHEET
Abdominal and lower limb arteries

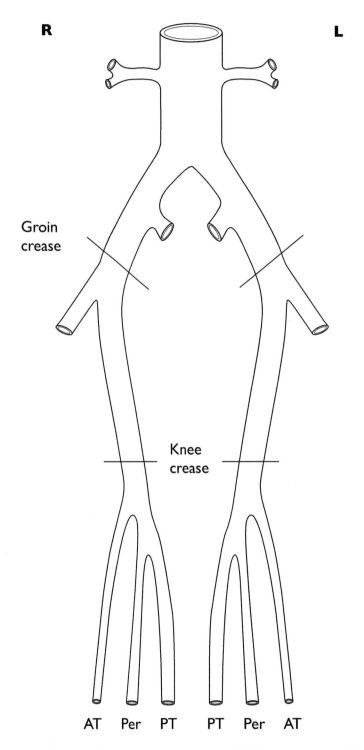

- Draw representation of plaque type and location, highlighting areas and degrees of stenoses.
- Draw representation of occlusions and their locations.
- Draw representation of aneurysm measurements and locations.
- Draw representations of stents and grafts.

7 RENOVASCULAR DISEASES

Ultrasound is used to screen for renovascular disease, help plan for treatment and follow the outcome. Even experienced sonographers detect only 80–90% of renal arteries. Accessory renal arteries are not always reliably detected by ultrasound and may be better shown by computed tomography angiography (CTA) or magnetic resonance angiography (MRA). Duplex scanning has 95% sensitivity and 90% specificity when compared with digital subtraction angiography (DSA) for detecting renal artery stenosis. However, contrast for DSA can worsen renal function. CTA or MRA may be preferred if ultrasound is inadequate.

ANATOMY

Vessels scanned for reporting:
- Aorta
- Renal arteries and veins
- Segmental, interlobar, interlobular, and arcuate arteries.

Other vessels discussed:
- Superior mesenteric artery – SMA
- Inferior mesenteric artery – IMA
- Common iliac artery – CIA
- Internal iliac artery – IIA
- External iliac artery – EIA
- Inferior vena cava – IVC.

Renal arteries (Fig. 7.1)
- Paired at approximately the same level at the first to second lumbar vertebrae.
- Arise at approximately right angles to the aorta, the left more posterior than the right.
- Each passes from the aorta to the renal hilum in the retroperitoneal plane just distal to the SMA.
- The right renal artery is longer than the left and usually passes posterior to the IVC.

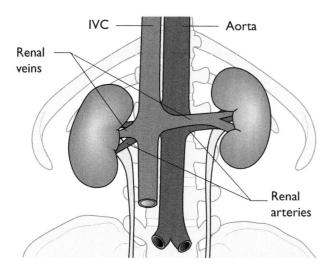

Fig. 7.1 *Renal arteries and veins.*

- The left renal artery has a more horizontal course to the kidney.
- Rare variations of their origins are as follows:
  - From a common stem.
  - Multiple from the aorta at different levels, each passing to the hilum.
  - From the CIA, IIA, or IMA.

Branches of the renal arteries (Fig. 7.2)
- Each divides into anterior and posterior branches near the hilum.

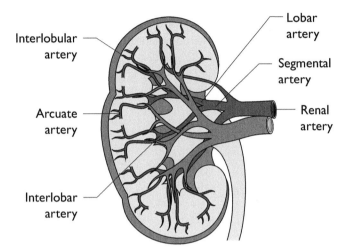

Fig. 7.2 *Branches of the renal artery.*

- The anterior branch divides into the apical, upper, middle and lower segmental branches, and the posterior branch continues on to supply the posterior aspect of the kidney.
- Segmental arteries become lobar arteries which branch into interlobar arteries between the renal pyramids.
- These terminate as arcuate arteries which course between the cortex and medulla.
- Arcuate arteries give off interlobular arteries which terminate as glomerular arterioles.

Accessory renal arteries (Fig. 7.3)
- 'End-arteries' pass directly to a segment of kidney other than the hilum.

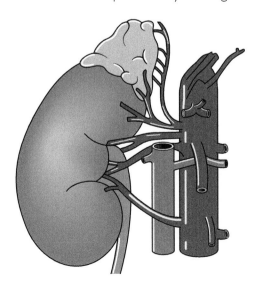

Fig. 7.3 *Accessory renal arteries.*

- They occur in 25–30% of individuals.
- They present on one or both sides, more often on the left than the right.
- They are more common above than below the main renal artery.
- Accessory arteries to the right kidney may pass in front of the IVC.
- They can arise from other aortic branches such as the SMA or CIA.

Renal veins (see Fig. 7.1)
- They pass to the IVC.
- They lie anterior to the renal arteries.
- The left renal vein is longer than the right and passes to the IVC between the aorta and the SMA.
- Tributaries are the left gonadal, adrenal and posterior lumbar veins.

Kidneys
- The right kidney is usually slightly lower and shorter than the left.
- Occasionally, they are considerably lower in the abdomen or pelvis than their normal position in the mid-abdomen.
- They can be fused, particularly at the lower poles to form a 'horseshoe kidney'.
- There may be only one kidney.

CLINICAL ASPECTS

Regional pathology
Renal artery stenosis or occlusion
- Renal artery stenosis or occlusion is most frequently due to atherosclerosis (Fig. 7.4):
  - It usually presents in older males.
  - It frequently leads to impaired renal function.
  - It usually affects the ostium or proximal renal artery.

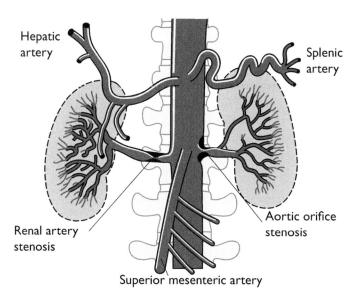

Hepatic artery

Splenic artery

Renal artery stenosis

Aortic orifice stenosis

Superior mesenteric artery

Fig. 7.4 *Renal artery stenoses from atherosclerosis.*
- *Right: plaque in the proximal renal artery (right kidney). Left: ostial stenosis from plaque in the adjacent aorta (left kidney).*

Adapted from Fig. 12.1d, Myers KA, Marshall RD, Freidin J. Principles of Pathology. Oxford: Blackwell, 1980. Reproduced with permission from Blackwell.

- Less frequently, stenosis is due to fibromuscular dysplasia (Fig. 7.5):
  - ○ It usually affects younger females.
  - ○ It rarely progresses to cause impaired renal function.
  - ○ It usually affects the mid to distal renal artery.
- Decreased renal perfusion from renal artery stenosis or occlusion can cause release of renin from endocrine cells in the glomeruli.
- Renin is part of a feedback loop that regulates arterial blood pressure by converting angiotensinogens to angiotensins which increase systemic peripheral resistance.
- In addition, an angiotensin acts at the adrenal gland to stimulate aldosterone secretion causing sodium and fluid retention.
- These effects can lead to secondary hypertension.

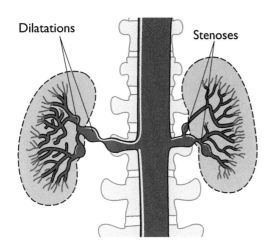

Fig. 7.5 *Renal artery stenoses from fibromuscular dysplasia.*
- *Multiple stenoses and dilations in mid to distal extrarenal arteries.*

Adapted from Fig. 12.1, Myers KA, Marshall RD, Freidin J. Principles of Pathology. Oxford: Blackwell, 1980. Reproduced with permission from Blackwell.

Renal artery aneurysms
- These occur in approximately 0.1% of individuals.
- Two-thirds are single and one-third multiple.
- They are bilateral in 20% of patients.
- The most frequent sites are in the main renal artery or at the bifurcation.
- Most are saccular.
- One-third are calcified.

Renal vein thrombosis
- Thrombosis of one or both renal veins or adjacent IVC can be spontaneous, secondary to hematological disturbance or from extension of a renal carcinoma.
- A retroperitoneal tumor or lymphadenopathy can cause extrinsic compression.
- The left renal vein can be compressed between the aorta and the SMA – the *'nutcracker syndrome'*.

Renal failure
- There may be acute renal injury or chronic renal disease.
- Decrease in glomerular filtration leads to failure to adequately filter waste products from the blood.
- Renal failure develops when the amount of functioning renal tissue is reduced by approximately 80%.
- Prerenal causes include the following:
  - Acute renal injury.
  - Renal trauma.
  - Loss of circulation from general trauma or shock.
  - Renal artery thrombosis.
  - Renal vein thrombosis.
- Intrinsic causes include the following:
  - Acute toxic injuries:
    - Drug overdose, e.g. aspirin.
    - Damage by medications, e.g. antibiotics.
    - Crush injury with toxic breakdown products.
  - Diabetic nephropathy.
  - Hypertensive nephropathy.
  - Polycystic kidney disease.
  - Glomerulonephritis, acute tubular necrosis or acute interstitial nephritis.
- Postrenal causes include the following:
  - Obstruction of the urinary tract.

Nephrotic syndrome
- This is a non-specific condition affecting renal tubules.
- The condition allows excessive leakage of plasma albumin but not red blood cells.
- Decreased serum albumin levels cause fluid and sodium retention leading to generalized edema.
- Secondary renal vein thrombosis can occur.

Clinical presentations
Renovascular hypertension
- Renal artery disease is frequently asymptomatic.
- If severe, it can lead to secondary renal hypertension.

Renal artery aneurysm
- It is usually asymptomatic and discovered by accident (DSA, CT, or MRI or with a plain radiograph if calcified).
- It may be associated with renal hypertension.
- Presentation can be with rupture.

Acute renal vein thrombosis
- Presentation may be with a painful mass in the flank, hematuria or thrombocytopenia.

Renal failure
- There may be few if any symptoms.
- Advanced disease is associated with vomiting, diarrhea, urinary symptoms and decreased urine flow.
- There is blood and/or protein in the urine, disturbed serum electrolytes and increased blood creatinine and urea levels.
- Fluid retention occurs.
- Patients may present with complications.

Nephrotic syndrome
- There is generalized edema, pleural effusions, pulmonary edema and ascites.
- Biochemical studies show decreased serum albumin, increased serum cholesterol and proteinuria.

Differential diagnosis – renal hypertension
- Essential (primary) hypertension.
- Coarctation of the suprarenal aorta.
- Adrenal gland tumors.

Treatment
Renovascular hypertension
- Initial management is by drug treatment.
- Intervention is required if hypertension remains uncontrolled or if there is progressive deterioration of renal function.
- In the past, this led to surgical endarterectomy or bypass grafting.
- Intervention for renal artery stenosis is now by balloon dilatation and stenting.
- Nephrectomy is performed if the kidney is infarcted or small and atrophic.

Renal artery aneurysm
- Observation if <1.5 cm diameter.
- Coil embolization or endoluminal stent-grafting.
- Arterial reconstruction in situ, or ex situ with removal of the kidney, followed by repair then reimplantation.
- Nephrectomy if large and inaccessible or for rupture.

Renal vein thrombosis
- Thrombolysis if detected early.
- Anticoagulation.
- Treatment of renal failure.

Renal failure
- Treatment of the underlying cause.
- Supportive medical treatment.
- Initial treatment is by peritoneal dialysis or hemodialysis (see Chapter 13).
- Kidney transplantation is indicated for irreversible renal failure (Fig. 7.6):
  - The kidney is placed in the iliac fossa.
  - The renal artery is anastomosed end to end to the IIA or end to side to the CIA, EIA, or aorta.
  - Anastomosis of the renal vein to an iliac vein.

Nephrotic syndrome
- General medical treatment.

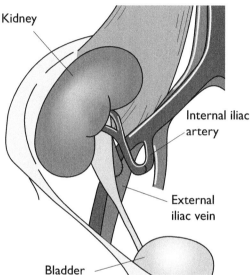

Fig. 7.6 *Kidney transplantation.*

Redrawn from Fig. P457, Scott R. Urology Illustrated. Oxford: Elsevier, 1982. © 1982 with permission from Elsevier.

WHAT DOCTORS NEED TO KNOW
- Is there disease in the renal arteries and what is its location and severity?
- Is renal artery disease atherosclerotic or due to fibromuscular dysplasia?
- Is the renal vein thrombosed?
- Is a stenosis within the proximal renal artery or at the renal artery ostium?
- Is there parenchymal disease of the kidneys and what is its severity?
- Is parenchymal disease focal or diffuse?
- Are there ultrasound changes over time with surveillance for untreated disease?
- Are there ultrasound changes with surveillance after renal artery balloon dilatation and stenting or kidney transplantation?

THE DUPLEX SCAN

Abbreviations
- Peak systolic velocity (cm/s) – PSV
- Renal:aortic ratio – RAR = $PSV_{Renal\ artery}/PSV_{Aorta}$
- End-diastolic velocity (cm/s) – EDV
- Resistance index – RI = (PSV – EDV)/PSV
- End-diastolic ratio – EDR = EDV/PSV
- Early systolic peak – ESP
- Acceleration time – AT = time from onset to ESP.

Indications for scanning

High-suspicion renal hypertension
- Uncontrolled hypertension.
- Hypertension in young patients.
- Hypertension of rapid onset.
- Epigastric or flank bruit.

Assessment before balloon dilatation and stenting
- Determine whether renal artery stenosis is at the ostium or in the proximal renal artery.
- Attempt to detect accessory renal arteries (Fig. 7.7).
- Determine whether there is parenchymal disease.

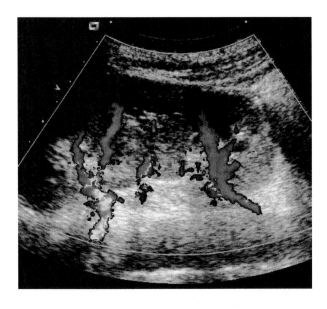

Fig. 7.7 *Color Doppler demonstrating an accessory renal artery.*
Image kindly supplied by Martin Necas, Hamilton, New Zealand.

Assessment before kidney transplantation
- Ensure that there is no disease in the aorta, IVC and iliac arteries and veins and that they are of adequate diameter.

Surveillance after balloon dilatation and stenting
- There is a poor correlation between restenosis and blood pressure control or deterioration of renal function.
- Scan post-treatment at 1 and 6 months and then annually.

Assessment after kidney transplantation (Fig. 7.8)

- Look for vascular abnormalities – renal artery or vein stenosis, thrombosis or compression or false aneurysm.
- Look for functional abnormalities – ischemic nephropathy causing acute tubular necrosis, acute and chronic rejection or ciclosporin (cyclosporin)-induced nephropathy.
- Look for morphological abnormalities – hydronephrosis or perirenal collections.

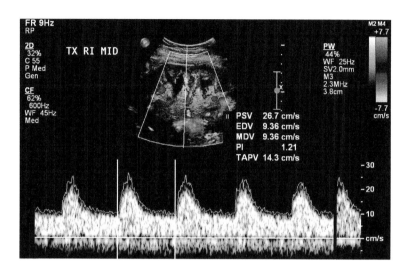

Fig. 7.8 *Color and spectral Doppler demonstration of a normal kidney transplant.*

Image kindly supplied by Martin Necas, Hamilton, New Zealand.

Normal findings

Normal waveforms for renal and intrarenal vessels

- *Renal artery*: it supplies low-resistance end-organs so waveforms have a blunted peak at systole and constant forward diastolic flow:
  - There is spectral broadening if a wide sample volume is used.
  - PSV decreases as the renal arteries and branches are followed out to the kidneys.
- *Renal vein*: it has flow towards the IVC with some respiratory and cardiac fluctuations.

Renal artery

- PSV 50–150 cm/s
- RAR 0.5–1.5
- EDV <50 cm/s

Renal artery at the hilum

- AT <100 ms

Intrarenal vessels

- EDR >0.30
- RI <70

The kidney – B-mode

- Pole-to-pole length ≥9 cm
- Width 4.5–6 cm
- Cortical thickness 1–2 cm

Criteria for diagnosing disease

● There is no consensus as to the best criteria for detecting critical renal artery stenosis or parenchymal disease.
● False-negative results may occur with fibromuscular dysplasia, branch artery stenoses, multiple renal arteries or impaired renal function.

Renal artery stenosis >60%

● RAR is preferred to PSV criteria.
● AT and RI (Fig. 7.9):
  ○ Easier to measure than PSV because they are not angle specific.
  ○ Helpful if proximal renal artery is obscured by bowel gas.
  ○ Have lower sensitivity for detecting renal artery disease.
  ○ Cannot distinguish proximal severe stenosis from occlusion.
  ○ Cannot detect proximal low-grade stenosis.

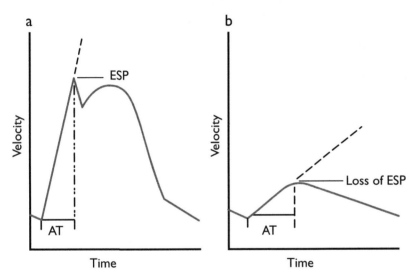

Fig. 7.9 *Calculation of the renal artery acceleration time (AT) to the early systolic peak (ESP):*
a Normal signal.
b The tardus–parvus renal artery signal (tardus – slowed systolic acceleration; parvus – low-amplitude systolic peak) with renal artery stenosis with loss of ESP.

Reprinted from Fig. 2, Lavoipierre AM, Dowling AJ, Little AF. Ultrasound of the renal vasculature. Ultrasound Quarterly 2000;**16**:123–132 with permission from Lippincott, Williams & Wilkins, Philadelphia.

Direct criteria in renal artery (Fig 7.10)
● RAR:
  ○ Highly specific – RAR >3.5
  ○ Highly sensitive – RAR >1.5
  ○ Compromise – RAR >2
● PSV:
  ○ Highly specific – PSV >220 cm/s
  ○ Highly sensitive – PSV >180 cm/s
  ○ Compromise – PSV >200 cm/s
● Post-stenotic turbulence.

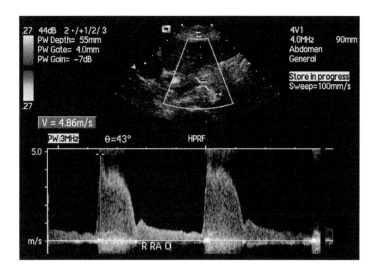

Fig. 7.10 *Spectral Doppler demonstrating >60% stenosis of the origin of the right renal artery.*

Image kindly supplied by Martin Necas, Hamilton, New Zealand.

Indirect criteria in the intrarenal arteries

- AT >100 ms
- RI >70
- *'Tardus parvus'* waveform (Fig. 7.11):
  - Pulsus tardus:
    - Prolonged systolic acceleration.
    - Delayed systolic upstroke.
    - Rounded systolic peak.
  - Pulsus parvus:
    - Diminished PSV.
- Loss of the ESP.

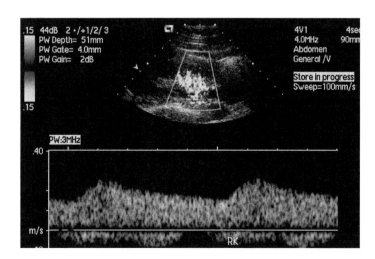

Fig. 7.11 *Spectral Doppler demonstrating a tardus parvus signal in intrarenal arteries distal to a renal artery stenosis.*

Image kindly supplied by Martin Necas, Hamilton, New Zealand.

PITFALL!

- The AT may be normal even with a proximal renal artery stenosis if there is high resistance due to associated intrarenal disease.

Renal artery stenosis <60%
Direct criteria in renal artery
- PSV >180 cm/s
- RAR 1.5 to <3.5
- No post-stenotic turbulence.

Renal artery occlusion
- A clear view of the renal artery with no flow detected with color or spectral Doppler.
- Reduced parenchymal renal blood flow velocity <10 cm/s.
- AT >100 ms in intrarenal arteries.
- Kidney length <9 cm.
- Collateral flow.

Parenchymal disease
- The EDR can assess the severity of intrarenal disease. EDR <0.3 predicts poor outcome post-revascularization.
- The preoperative RI predicts improvement of blood pressure and renal function after renal artery balloon dilation or stenting – RI >80 indicates that treatment may be ineffective and RI <80 predicts a good response.

Criteria
- B-mode appearance of kidney:
  - Pole-to-pole length <9 cm:
    - Right kidney >2.5 cm smaller than left kidney.
    - Left kidney >1.5 cm smaller than right kidney.
  - Cortical hyperechogenicity on the B-scan.
- Intrarenal Doppler characteristics:
  - EDR reduction:
    - 0.25–0.30 – minor disease.
    - 0.20–0.25 – moderate disease.
    - <0.20 – severe disease.
  - RI >80.
  - RI >5% difference for a unilateral stenosis compared with the other side.
- Cortical thickness <1 cm.

PITFALL!
- Measurement of kidney length with ultrasound is imprecise and can be difficult to reproduce.

Fibromuscular dysplasia

- 'String of beads' appearance on ultrasound (Fig 7.12).
- Associated stenoses present.

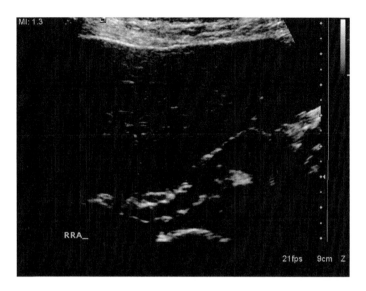

Fig. 7.12 B-mode image of fibromuscular dysplasia in mid-right renal artery.

Image kindly supplied by Martin Necas, Hamilton, New Zealand.

Renal vein thrombosis

- The renal vein is seen but no color or spectral Doppler signal is detected.
- B-mode shows echogenic material filling the lumen.
- Color Doppler shows intraluminal filling defect.
- There is a lack of venous flow in the parenchyma, an enlarged kidney and dilated intrarenal veins and venous collaterals.
- There is high resistance flow with reversed flow in diastole in the renal artery (Fig. 7.13).
- There is increased distal renal vein diameter if compressed by the 'nutcracker syndrome'.

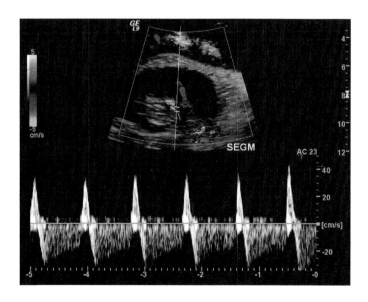

Fig. 7.13 Spectral Doppler showing to-and-fro flow in an intrarenal artery, indicating renal vein thrombosis.

Image kindly supplied by Martin Necas, Hamilton, New Zealand.

Thromboembolism from renal artery (Fig 7.14)

- Color Doppler can demonstrate a lack of flow in the renal parenchyma caused by thromboembolism lodged in the intrarenal arteries.

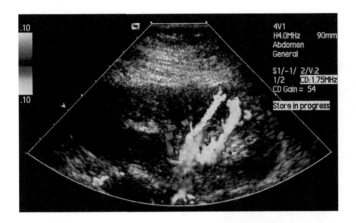

Fig. 7.14 *Color Doppler demonstrating lack of flow in kidney parenchyma due to thromboembolism.*

Image kindly supplied by Martin Necas, Hamilton, New Zealand.

Kidney transplantation complications

- Ultrasound can screen for problems that are not yet clinically obvious or detect reasons for deteriorating renal function.
- Renal artery stenosis is most common from 3 months to 2 years post-transplantation.
- Renal artery stenosis is most commonly at approximately 1 cm distal to the anastomosis site due to surgical clamping.
- A renal artery/common iliac artery PSV ratio >3.0 with post-stenotic turbulence is diagnostic for >60% of cases of renal artery stenosis.
- RI <0.6 in the intrarenal arteries can suggest a more proximal renal artery stenosis.
- RI >0.7 in the intrarenal arteries can suggest transplant rejection or renal vein thrombosis.
- Increasing RI, decreased diastolic flow and decreasing EDR with serial studies may indicate acute tubular necrosis, transplant rejection or ciclosporin (cyclosporin) toxicity before clinical features become apparent.
- A falling RI is a good sign that acute tubular necrosis or rejection is recovering.
- Transplanted renal vein thrombosis shows the same ultrasound appearances as a thrombosed native renal vein.

PROTOCOLS FOR SCANNING

- Preparing the patient, selecting the best transducer and general principles for scanning are discussed in Chapter 3 (pages 40–42).
- For renal vessel studies, prepare the patient nil orally until 1 hour before the scan after which several glasses of water are taken.

TIPS!

- Power Doppler provides greater sensitivity for intrarenal vessels but is subject to flash artifact.
- Harmonic imaging aids B-mode identification of the renal arteries and kidneys.

Aorta
Position the patient and select windows
- Scan with the patient lying supine. Image from the anterior approach through rectus abdominis to the left of midline and superior to the umbilicus.
- Turn the patient to right lateral decubitus position and use a coronal (flank) window if the patient is gassy or obese.
- Tilt the table at various angles to shift gas to different positions in the bowel and to let the bowel descend.
- Use the transducer to massage the abdomen from lateral to medial to manipulate bowel gas.

Scan the aorta
- Commence imaging at the xiphoid process in longitudinal to evaluate the full length of the abdominal aorta. Note tortuosity, aneurysmal dilation or arterial wall irregularity. Perform a full scan for an abdominal aortic aneurysm if detected (see Chapter 6).
- Record sample spectral traces throughout the aorta. Record PSV in the suprarenal aorta at the level of the SMA in longitudinal to calculate the RAR.
- Image the aorta in transverse and work down to the left renal vein as it crosses anterior to the aorta and posterior to the SMA which is a reliable landmark to locate the renal arteries. The right renal artery is located at approximately 10 o'clock and the left renal artery at approximately 4 o'clock.

Proximal to mid-renal arteries and veins
Position the patient and select windows
- Keep the patient positioned as for the aorta. The renal arteries can be clearly identified in B-mode but Doppler angles >60° may make this position unsuitable.
- Roll the patient in a semi-lateral decubitus position and angle the transducer away from the midline in the oblique approach. It should be possible to insonate the appropriate proximal to mid-renal artery with Doppler angles of 45–60°.

Scan the proximal to mid-renal arteries and veins
- Increase the sweep speed to better define the systolic upstroke.
- Use color Doppler to identify each renal artery as it arises from the lateral wall of the aorta just distal to the left renal vein.
- Begin in the aorta, keep the sample volume small, ask the patient to stop breathing for short intervals and 'walk' the spectral Doppler sample volume through the orifice of each renal artery and along its length for as far as you can image; pay particular attention to any areas of color aliasing.
- Record sample traces and PSV at the origin, proximal and mid segments or wherever a stenosis is detected.
- Calculate the RAR.
- Use B-mode to identify a renal artery stent; walk the spectral Doppler sample through the stent to obtain PSV and a sample spectral trace.
- With B-mode and color Doppler look for multiple renal arteries.
- Scan for renal vein thrombosis demonstrating no color or spectral trace in the vein.
- Look for 'nutcracker syndrome' with compression between the SMA and aorta and distal renal vein dilation.

Distal renal artery and vein, intrarenal arteries and kidney
Position the patient and select windows

- Position the patient in lateral decubitus and image from a coronal (flank) window.
- An intercostal view through the ribs on a deep inspiration is helpful.
- Tilt the bed in reverse Trendelenburg* to help the kidneys descend.
- Less commonly, lay the patient prone or in lateral decubitus and image from a posterior window.

Scan the distal renal artery and vein, intrarenal arteries and kidney

- In longitudinal, measure the pole-to-pole kidney length (Fig. 7.15). Look for increased cortical echogenicity and cortical thinning.
- Use color or power Doppler to note good perfusion throughout the kidney.
- Use color or power Doppler to identify the renal artery entering the hilum and the subsequent branches. Make the sample volume large and turn off the angle facility because the only concern now is with Doppler waveform morphology and not velocities.
- Look for multiple renal arteries with B-mode and color Doppler in both transverse and longitudinal. If the main renal artery is noted to enter the kidney eccentrically, this may indicate an accessory renal artery.
- Increase the sweep speed to better define the systolic upstroke and reduce spectral pulse repetition frequency (PRF) so that waveforms nearly fill the entire scale.
- Ask the patient to hold a breath to obtain waveforms from segmental arteries and interlobar arteries. Do not take sample traces in the arcuate arteries because they lie perpendicular to the transducer and will produce weak Doppler signals.
- Use the advanced measurements facility to calculate AT at the hilum. Calculate the EDR and RI from representative segmental and interlobar arteries.
- Note non-vascular abnormalities such as cysts, tumors, hydronephrosis or calculi.
- It may be possible to trace the renal artery back to its origin with the aorta.
- Trace the renal vein back to the IVC, scanning for renal vein thrombosis and demonstrating no color or spectral trace in the vein.

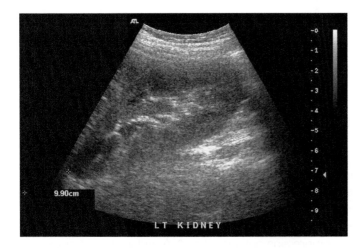

Fig. 7.15 B-mode image of kidney in longitudinal.

---

*Friedrich Trendelenburg, 1844–1924, German surgeon

Kidney transplant
Position the patient and select windows
● Lay the patient supine and scan through the appropriate iliac fossa.
● Lay the patient in lateral decubitus and scan through the coronal (flank) window.

Scan a kidney transplant
● Trace the renal artery from the anastomosis and then continue to examine as for a native renal artery study.
● Determine patency and record PSV in the main renal artery, at the anastomosis site and in the proximal native iliac artery.
● Calculate the renal artery/common iliac artery PSV ratio.
● Note that end-to-side anastomosis can cause turbulence without increased velocities.
● Examine the whole kidney in color or power Doppler to detect a focal or global decrease in parenchymal vascularity.
● Calculate RI from the segmental and interlobar arteries of the upper, mid and lower portions of the transplant.
● Determine patency of the transposed renal vein.
● Use B-mode to measure kidney length and show hydronephrosis or perirenal fluid collections.

ULTRASOUND IMAGES TO RECORD
Assessment of native renal arteries and kidneys
● Sample spectral traces to record PSV and EDV of the suprarenal aorta, both renal arteries in proximal, mid and distal segments, renal arteries at the hilum, and segmental and interlobar arteries.
● If present, sample spectral trace in stent and note the RAR.
● RAR of the proximal renal arteries.

- AT in the renal arteries at the hila.
- Note presence of accessory renal arteries.
- EDR and RI for representative segmental and interlobar arteries.
- Sample spectral traces of both renal veins if clinical indication is present.
- Spectral trace within thrombosed renal vein.
- Spectral traces proximal to, within and distal to sites of stenosis; note the extent and location from the renal artery origin and in particular if a proximal or ostial stenosis.
- B-mode image of each kidney length (two to three measurements to calculate average result).
- Power or color Doppler image to demonstrate renal perfusion.
- Other pathology such as fibromuscular dysplasia, a renal cyst, or calculus, or an abdominal aortic aneurysm.

Assessment before kidney transplantation

- Determine patency of IVC and bilateral common, internal and external iliac veins.
- Measure diameters and note disease of aorta and bilateral common, internal and external iliac arteries.

Surveillance of kidney transplantation

- B-mode image of kidney length, width, and cortical thickness.
- Sample spectral traces of native iliac artery both proximal to and at the anastomosis site, and within the proximal transposed renal artery.
- RAR of transposed renal artery.
- Sample spectral trace of transposed renal vein.
- AT of renal artery at hilum.
- Sample spectral traces and RI of representative segmental and interlobar arteries.

WORKSHEET
Renal artery studies

R   L

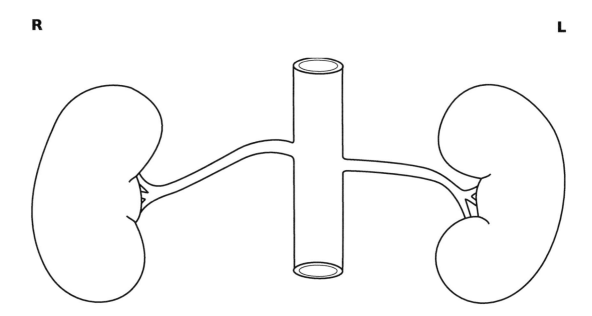

- Draw representation of plaque type and location, highlighting areas and degrees of stenoses.
- Draw representations of occlusions and their locations.
- Draw representations of stents.
- Draw representation of thrombus and location.

8 CELIAC AND MESENTERIC ARTERIAL DISEASES

Atherosclerosis is not as common in these arteries as at other sites. Disease usually involves their origins and can be demonstrated by duplex scanning in more than 90% of patients. There are non-atherosclerotic arterial diseases that have characteristic ultrasound features. Duplex scanning can detect disease, plan for intervention and follow results of treatment. However, it is usually necessary to confirm disease by angiography.

ANATOMY

Arteries scanned for reporting:
- Abdominal aorta
- Celiac axis
- Splenic artery
- Common and proper hepatic arteries
- Left gastric artery
- Superior mesenteric artery – SMA
- Inferior mesenteric artery – IMA.

Other vessels discussed or seldom scanned:
- Right, middle and left hepatic arteries
- Right gastric artery
- Cystic artery
- Gastroduodenal artery
- Pancreatic branches
- Inferior pancreaticoduodenal artery
- Middle, left and right colic arteries
- Ileocolic artery
- Jejunal arteries
- Ileal arteries
- Sigmoid branches
- Superior rectal artery
- Left renal vein
- Portal vein.

- The three main arterial branches to the gastrointestinal that track from the anterior aspect of the abdominal aorta from proximal to distal are the celiac axis, SMA and IMA.

Celiac axis (Fig. 8.1)

- It is the first major branch of the abdominal aorta.
- It supplies the liver, stomach, spleen, gallbladder and pancreas.
- It divides into the splenic, common hepatic and left gastric arteries at 1–2 cm from its origin.
- The splenic artery is the largest, located superior and anterior to the splenic vein.
- The splenic artery gives off pancreatic branches.
- The common hepatic artery divides into the proper hepatic and gastroduodenal arteries.
- The proper hepatic artery tracks next to the portal vein and common bile duct (CBD) to form the portal triad.
- The proper hepatic artery gives off the right gastric artery which supplies the inferior part of the stomach.
- The proper hepatic artery divides into right and left branches which enter the liver at the porta hepatis and lie adjacent to the right and left portal veins.
- The right hepatic artery is the main supply to the bile duct and gives off the cystic artery to the gallbladder.
- The left gastric artery is the smallest and supplies part of the stomach.

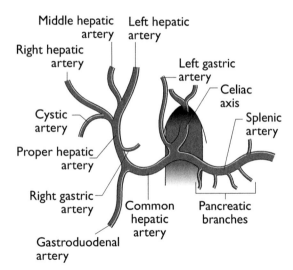

Fig. 8.1 *The celiac axis and its branches.*

SMA (Fig. 8.2)

- The origin is 1–2 cm distal to the celiac axis and tracks right of the midline.
- It supplies the distal duodenum, small intestine and ascending and transverse colon.
- The proximal segment lies parallel to the aorta between the pancreas and the left renal vein.
- It lies to the left of the superior mesenteric vein, posterior to the splenic and portal veins and anterior to the left renal vein.
- The origin is surrounded by an echogenic fat pad.
- It normally gives rise to the inferior pancreaticoduodenal, middle colic, right colic, ileocolic, jejunal and ileal arteries.

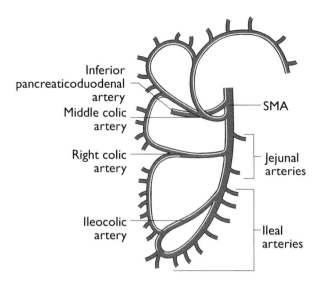

Inferior pancreaticoduodenal artery

Middle colic artery

Right colic artery

Ileocolic artery

SMA

Jejunal arteries

Ileal arteries

Fig. 8.2 *The SMA and its branches.*

IMA (Fig. 8.3)

- The origin is 3–5 cm proximal to the aortic bifurcation and tracks left of the midline.
- It supplies the descending and sigmoid colon and upper rectum.
- It normally gives the left colic, sigmoid and superior rectal arteries.

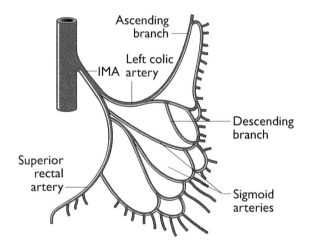

Ascending branch

Left colic artery

IMA

Descending branch

Superior rectal artery

Sigmoid arteries

Fig. 8.3 *The IMA and its branches.*
Redrawn from Fig. 19.1, Strandness DE. Collateral Circulation in Clinical Surgery. Philadelphia: WB Saunders, 1969. Reproduced with permission.

Anatomical variations
Common trunks

- There is a common trunk for the celiac axis and SMA in 3% of individuals.
- The IMA and SMA may have a common trunk.
- A common origin for the SMA and common hepatic artery from the aorta is rare.
- The middle and right colic arteries may have a common stem.

Hepatic artery
- The anatomy for the common hepatic artery and branches shown in Fig. 8.1 is present in two-thirds of individuals.
- Variations can affect techniques for liver transplantation and catheterization for tumor embolization.
- The common hepatic artery can arise from the SMA or the aorta.
- The right hepatic artery can arise from the SMA (10–20%):
  - It usually passes lateral and behind the portal vein.
  - It can pass behind or through the head of the pancreas.
- The left hepatic artery can arise from the left gastric artery (3–10%).
- There can be an accessory right or left hepatic artery arising from the SMA or left gastric arteries respectively.
- Accordingly, there can be up to four hepatic arteries.
- The middle hepatic artery can arise from any of the above arteries.

SMA
- Inconstant branches include the dorsal pancreatic, inferior pancreatic, right hepatic, common hepatic and accessory middle colic arteries.
- The IMA, splenic, gastroduodenal or cystic arteries can arise from the SMA.
- The middle colic artery may arise from the splenic artery or the IMA, or it may be absent.
- The left colic artery may be a branch of the SMA.
- The right colic artery may arise from the middle colic, ileocolic or left colic arteries, or it may be absent.
- The ileocolic artery may arise directly from the aorta.

Collaterals between the visceral arteries (Fig. 8.4)
- Celiac axis to SMA through the gastroduodenal and pancreaticoduodenal arteries.
- Middle colic branch of the SMA to the left colic branch of the IMA – the 'meandering mesenteric artery'.
- Ileocolic, and right, left and middle colic branches of the SMA to the left colic and sigmoid arteries of the IMA – the 'marginal artery of Drummond.'

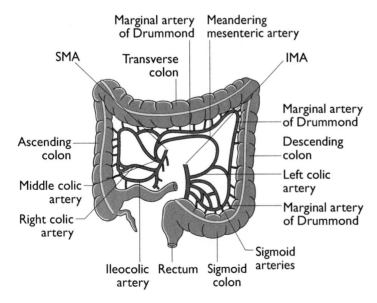

Fig. 8.4 Collaterals between the three main visceral arteries.

Redrawn from Fig. 24.2, Strandness DE. Collateral Circulation in Clinical Surgery. Philadelphia: WB Saunders, 1969. Reproduced with permission.

CLINICAL ASPECTS

Regional pathology

Chronic mesenteric ischemia (CMI)

- Stenosis or occlusion of the celiac or mesenteric arteries or their branches can cause CMI.
- It usually requires two or all three arteries to be affected by high-grade stenosis or occlusion to cause clinical symptoms because there is a rich collateral circulation.

Median arcuate ligament syndrome (MALS)

- The median arcuate ligament of the diaphragm is a fibrous arch that unites the diaphragmatic crura on either side of the aortic hiatus.
- It normally passes cranial to the origin of the celiac axis.
- It passes at the level of the origin of the celiac axis in 10–25% of individuals.
- This can lead to entrapment and compression of the celiac axis.
- Intermittent compression during expiration can damage the vessel wall, with deposition of thrombotic material causing permanent stenosis and subsequent post-stenotic dilation.

Acute mesenteric ischemia (AMI)

- The SMA can be acutely occluded by an embolus from the heart.
- Acute thrombosis of the SMA or more distal small arteries and veins can occur, commonly due to severe dehydration or thrombophilia, or as a complication of some therapeutic drugs.

Visceral artery aneurysms

- Visceral aneurysms are uncommon. In order of frequency they occur in the following arteries:
  - Splenic artery.
  - Hepatic artery.
  - SMA.
  - Celiac axis.
  - Other branches.
- Aneurysms are usually detected incidentally from wall calcification seen with plain radiograph or by ultrasound, CT or MRI.
- Ultrasound can distinguish an aneurysm from an abdominal cyst or tumor.

Clinical presentations and treatment

Chronic mesenteric ischemia

- CMI is considered in patients presenting with postprandial pain, weight loss and malabsorption, although these symptoms are usually due to other more common diseases.
- However, presentation can be with vague abdominal symptoms.
- An epigastric bruit is present.
- Treatment is by surgical reconstruction or endovascular stenting.

Median arcuate ligament syndrome

- Patients most commonly present with postprandial epigastric pain, weight loss and an epigastric bruit.
- This may require surgery to divide the median arcuate ligament.

Acute mesenteric ischemia

- Presentation of AMI is usually with abdominal pain, gastrointestinal bleeding, vomiting and diarrhea or as profound shock.
- Treatment is usually by surgical reconstruction or resection of infarcted bowel.

Visceral artery aneurysms

- Splenic artery aneurysms are unusual in that they are most often found in younger females and have a tendency to enlarge and rupture in the third trimester of pregnancy.
- They are usually asymptomatic until they present with rupture which is usually intraperitoneal and catastrophic.
- Treatment is by ligation, excision, bypass grafting or endovascular stent-grafting.

Differential diagnosis

- Other diseases are more likely to cause chronic or acute abdominal pain:
  - Appendicitis.
  - Cholecystitis.
  - Pancreatitis.
  - Peptic ulceration.
  - Renal colic.
  - Leaking or ruptured abdominal aortic aneurysm.

WHAT DOCTORS NEED TO KNOW

- Is there stenosis in the celiac axis, SMA or IMA, and how severe is it?
- Is there evidence of extrinsic compression of the celiac axis origin by the median arcuate ligament?
- Is there occlusion of one or more of the arteries or their branches?
- Is there an aneurysm of one of the arteries, where is it and what is its diameter?
- What is the flow direction in arteries that may act as collaterals, with stenosis or occlusion of the celiac axis or SMA?
- Are there anatomical variations?

THE DUPLEX SCAN

Abbreviations

- Peak systolic velocity (cm/s) – PSV.
- End-diastolic velocity (cm/s) – EDV.

Indications for scanning

- Suspected CMI.
- To demonstrate MALS.
- To detect a visceral artery aneurysm.
- To monitor known arterial stenosis.
- For follow-up after intervention for stenotic disease.
- Doppler ultrasound is not usually performed for AMI due to its rapid onset and the need for urgent surgery.

Normal arterial flow
Celiac axis

- The celiac axis and its major branches show similar low-resistance flow patterns of monophasic waveforms with a sharp systolic upstroke and a relatively large diastolic component consistent with flow into the liver and spleen and PSV <200 cm/s (Fig. 8.5).
- Taking food does not affect the flow.
- The left gastric artery is rarely seen with ultrasound.
- The splenic artery may show turbulent flow due to tortuosity.

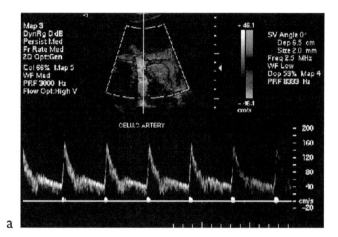

Fig. 8.5 *Normal celiac axis:*
a Spectral Doppler.
b Color Doppler.
- *Note the bifurcation forming the hepatic and splenic arteries to produce the 'seagull sign.'*

SMA

- The flow pattern varies according to the metabolic activity of the intestine (Fig. 8.6).
- In the fasting state, the SMA normally exhibits a high-resistance pattern with a sharp systolic upstroke and variable diastolic component with low forward flow, reversed flow or both, and the PSV is <275 cm/s and usually between 100 and 140 cm/s.
- After ingesting a meal, there is normally a considerable increase in SMA blood flow over 20–30 min, a fall in resistance, a threefold increase in EDV and an increase in arterial diameter.

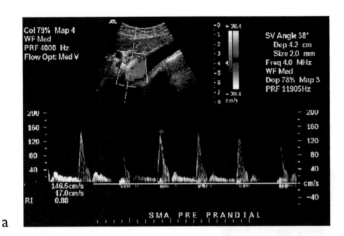

a

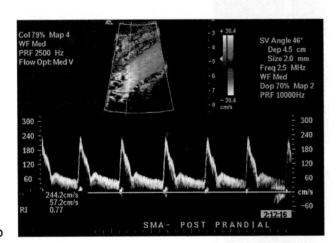

b

Fig. 8.6 Normal SMA – spectral waveforms:
- **a** High-resistance signal in the fasting state.
- **b** Increased velocities with high diastolic velocities and absence of reverse flow after a standard meal.

Anatomical variations

- If there is a common trunk for the celiac axis and SMA, there will be a low-resistance signal at the origin of the trunk changing to a high-resistance signal in the SMA distal to the origins of the hepatic and splenic arteries.
- A low-resistance signal will also be present in the proximal SMA if the common or right hepatic artery arises from it more distally.
- There will be increased PSV in the hepatic artery if it is a branch of the SMA.

IMA

- If seen, the waveform is similar to the SMA with a high-resistance pattern but less reversed diastolic flow and lower velocities.
- IMA velocities are not likely to be affected by ingesting food.

Criteria for diagnosing disease

Celiac artery stenosis or occlusion (Fig. 8.7)

- Stenosis or occlusion usually affects the first 1–2 cm of the artery.
- Occlusion is associated with absent color Doppler images and loss of spectral signal.
- Retrograde flow in the left hepatic artery is diagnostic for severe celiac artery stenosis or occlusion.
- There may be retrograde flow in the common hepatic or splenic artery.
- Celiac axis stenosis due to MALS causes high PSVs during maximum expiration which disappear with deep inspiration or by standing the patient. The origin appears to be 'bent' upwards losing its straight orientation.
- Post-stenotic turbulence.

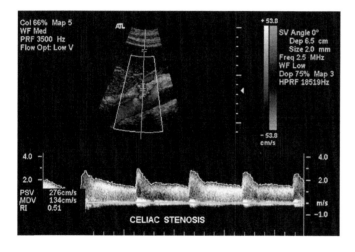

Fig. 8.7 *Spectral tracing for severe celiac artery stenosis.*

SMA stenosis or occlusion

- Stenosis or occlusion usually affects the proximal artery.
- Occlusion is associated with absent color Doppler images and loss of the spectral signal in the SMA.
- Retrograde flow may be seen in the first set of branches of the SMA feeding the more distal artery.
- Postprandial studies add little to the examination if the fasting PSV is raised.
- The decrease in PSV beyond an SMA stenosis or occlusion is less if there is a good collateral circulation feeding the SMA.
- A low-resistance Doppler signal in the IMA or B-mode evidence of dilation suggests that it is acting as a collateral for occlusive disease in the SMA or celiac axis.

- Criteria for stenosis for each have recently been updated*.
- Stenoses in native arteries have different thresholds to stenoses within stented arteries (*Table 8.1*).
- Post-stenotic turbulence.

Table 8.1 *Comparison of native and in-stent stenoses.*

	Native stenosis PSV (cm/s)	In-stent stenosis PSV (cm/s)
>50% stenosis		
Celiac axis	240	275
SMA	295	325
>70% stenosis		
Celiac axis	320	365
SMA	400	415

IMA stenosis or occlusion
- Stenosis or occlusion usually affects the proximal artery.
- IMA stenosis criteria are PSV >200 cm/s with post-stenotic turbulence.
- IMA occlusion is confirmed with loss of flow on color and spectral Doppler.

PROTOCOLS FOR SCANNING

- Preparing the patient, selecting the best transducer and general principles for scanning are discussed in Chapter 3 (pages 40–42).
- If a postprandial study is requested, give the patient a high-calorie high-protein drink (flavored milk) and biscuits and repeat scanning of the SMA after 20 min.

Position the patient and select windows
- Scan with the patient lying supine.
- Image from an anterior approach through rectus abdominis to the left of the midline, superior to the umbilicus and at the umbilical level.
- Turn the patient to right or left lateral decubitus position and use a coronal (flank) window if the patient is gassy or obese.
- Tilt the table at various angles to shift gas to different positions in the bowel.
- Use the transducer to massage the abdomen from lateral to medial to push bowel gas away.

Scan the aorta
- In transverse, identify the suprarenal aorta. It lies left of the inferior vena cava (IVC).
- In longitudinal, take a sample spectral trace and measure PSV and EDV above the level of the celiac axis.
- Use B-mode to help identify echogenic atherosclerosis.
- Examine for aortic aneurysm or atherosclerotic disease if present (see Chapter 6).

*AbuRahma *et al.* Duplex velocity criteria for native celiac/superior mesenteric stenosis vs in-stent stenosis. *J Vasc Surg*, 2012 Mar; **55**(2): 730-8

Scan the celiac axis

- In transverse with color Doppler, scan the abdominal midline looking for the celiac axis dividing into the hepatic and splenic arteries – the '*seagull sign*' (Fig. 8.5).
- Spectral traces of the celiac axis and hepatic and splenic arteries are taken with the transducer in transverse.
- Walk the spectral Doppler sample throughout all native or stented arteries to ensure that a focal increase in PSV indicated by color aliasing is not missed.
- Record PSV and EDV at the origin, the proximal trunk of the celiac axis and the bifurcation into hepatic and splenic arteries.
- Record PSV and EDV in the proximal common hepatic and splenic arteries.
- If MALS is suspected, take a specific note of external compression and reorientation of the proximal segment during maximum expiration. Take spectral traces and record the PSV with normal inspiration and maximum expiration or the patient standing.
- Take spectral traces proximal to, at and distal to each stenosis. Note the location from the anatomical landmark, the extent and the severity. Note the presence of post-stenotic turbulence.
- Take spectral traces proximal to, within and distal to the occlusions. Note the location from the anatomical landmark and the extent.
- With spectral Doppler, identify flow direction in arteries acting as collaterals.
- Use B-mode to help identify echogenic atherosclerosis.
- If there is an aneurysm, use B-mode to measure its proximal, maximum and distal diameters.
- Note the presence of mural thrombus and record the residual diameter. Record the location and length.

NOTE!

- It is helpful to evaluate the common hepatic artery if the celiac axis is difficult to identify or at an angle that makes it difficult to obtain accurate Doppler samples.

Scan the SMA

- With color Doppler in either transverse or longitudinal, identify the SMA arising from the anterior aorta at 1–2 cm distal to the celiac origin.
- In color Doppler and longitudinal, trace the SMA. It lies parallel and superficial to the aorta and it is usually possible to follow the artery for 5 cm.
- Spectral traces of the SMA are taken in longitudinal.
- Heel - toe the transducer tilting cranially to create a Doppler angle ≤60° in the proximal segment.
- Correct Doppler angles can be assisted by the patient taking an inspiration.
- 'Walk' the Doppler sample throughout the native or stented SMA to ensure that a focal increase in PSV indicated by color aliasing is not missed.
- Record PSV and EDV at the origin, proximal and distal SMA.
- Take spectral traces proximal to, at and distal to each stenosis. Note the location from the anatomical landmark, the extent and the severity. Note the presence of post-stenotic turbulence.
- Take spectral traces proximal and distal to occlusions. Note the location from the anatomical landmark and the extent.

- Take spectral traces proximal to, within and distal to occlusions. Note the location from the anatomical landmark and the extent.
- With spectral Doppler, identify flow direction in arteries acting as collaterals.
- Use B-mode to help identify echogenic atherosclerosis.
- If there is an aneurysm, use B-mode to measure its proximal, maximum and distal diameters.
- Note the presence of mural thrombus in the AAA, record the residual diameter and its location from an anatomical landmark, and length.
- If AMI is indicated, trace the smaller branches of the SMA. Look for loss of color and spectral Doppler indicating occlusion from embolus or thrombosis.

Scan the IMA

- This is less clinically relevant.
- Note whether the IMA is patent, occluded or not visualized.
- The IMA is more frequently seen in longitudinal than in transverse.
- If found in transverse, it is at about 12 to 2 o'clock from the aorta.
- The IMA may not be detected unless it is acting as a collateral with occlusive disease of the celiac axis or SMA or if the patient is thin.
- Spectral traces of the IMA are taken in longitudinal.
- Record PSV and EDV in the origin and proximal IMA.
- Take spectral traces proximal to, at and distal to each stenosis. Note the location from the anatomical landmark, the extent and the severity. Note the presence of post-stenotic turbulence.
- Take spectral traces proximal to, within and distal to occlusions. Note the location from an anatomical landmark and the extent.
- With spectral Doppler, identify flow direction in arteries acting as collaterals.
- Use B-mode to help identify echogenic atherosclerosis.
- If there is an aneurysm, use B-mode to measure its proximal, maximum and distal diameters.
- Note the presence of mural thrombus in the aneurysm and record the residual diameter. Record the location and length.

PITFALLS!

- As a result of anatomical variations, do not assume that an artery is occluded if it is not seen.
- Tortuosity of the celiac axis can make it difficult to obtain an accurate angle of insonation.
- Calcification can cause shadowing which may be incorrectly interpreted as an occlusion.
- Increased flow in a mesenteric artery as a compensatory mechanism can be incorrectly interpreted as being due to stenosis – always determine whether or not there is post-stenotic turbulence.
- A collateral adjacent to an occluded artery can be incorrectly interpreted as the normal artery.

ULTRASOUND IMAGES TO RECORD

CMI
- Sample spectral traces for each artery listed.
- Spectral traces proximal to, within and distal to each stenosis; note the location from anatomical landmark, the extent and the severity.
- Note post-stenotic turbulence.
- Spectral trace proximal to, within and distal to occlusions; note the location from the anatomical landmark and the extent.
- Note flow direction in arteries acting as collaterals.
- Note anatomical variations.
- Note waveform morphology in SMA.

MALS
- Sample spectral traces for each artery listed.
- Spectral traces and note PSV in the proximal celiac axis with normal inspiration, maximum expiration or the patient standing.
- Note if external compression and deviation of the proximal celiac axis with maximum expiration.
- Note post-stenotic turbulence.

Post-stent insertion
- Sample spectral traces for each artery listed.
- Spectral traces proximal to and within stented regions. Note the PSV.
- Note post-stenotic turbulence.

Aneurysms
- B-mode of length of aneurysm in longitudinal.
- B-mode of maximum transverse and anteroposterior diameters of aneurysm.
- B-mode of mural thrombus and residual lumen diameter of aneurysm.
- B-mode of proximal and distal diameters of adjacent normal artery.
- Note the location of the aneurysm.

Postprandial studies
- Spectral traces in the SMA pre- and postprandial.
- Note PSVs and post-stenotic turbulence.

WORKSHEET
Celiac and mesenteric arteries

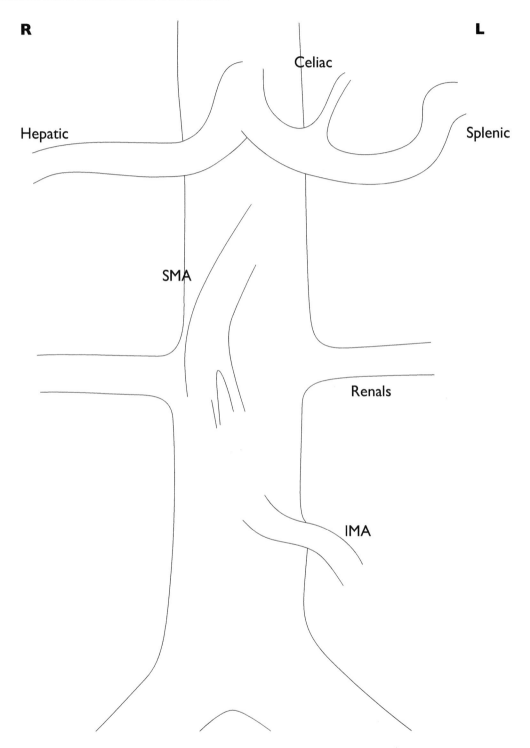

R   L

Celiac

Hepatic   Splenic

SMA

Renals

IMA

- Draw representation of plaque type and location, highlighting areas and degrees of stenoses.
- Draw representations of occlusions and their locations.
- Draw representations of stents.

9 HEPATOPORTAL VENOUS DISEASES

Intrinsic vascular disease or extrinsic vascular compression can cause obstruction of the extra- or intrahepatic portal or hepatic venous systems. Ultrasound is used to assess vascular changes, plan for interventional treatment and perform surveillance in patients with clinical features of chronic hepatic or splenic disease. Other investigations that may be required are endoscopy, transjugular measurement of the hepatic venous pressure gradient, transjugular or percutaneous liver biopsy under ultrasound guidance, computed tomography (CT), magnetic resonance imaging (MRI) and angiography.

ANATOMY

Vessels scanned for reporting:
- Portal vein
- Left and right portal veins
- Middle, left and right hepatic veins
- Inferior vena cava – IVC
- Splenic vein
- Superior mesenteric vein – SMV
- Inferior mesenteric vein – IMV
- Left renal vein
- Coronary (left gastric) vein
- Paraumbilical vein
- Hepatic artery
- Superior mesenteric artery – SMA
- Inferior mesenteric artery – IMA.

Portal veins, SMV and splenic vein (Fig. 9.1)
- Abdominal veins drain to the systemic IVC or portal venous system.
- The IMV does not follow the course of the IMA but drains into the splenic vein.

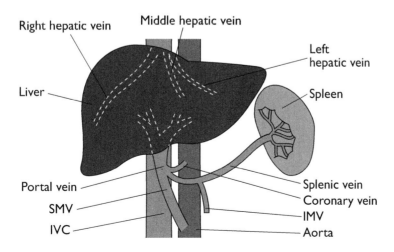

Fig. 9.1 Intra-abdominal systemic, portal and hepatic veins.

- The splenic vein and SMV join to form the portal vein.
- The SMV lies to the right of the SMA and anterior to the aorta.
- The portal vein lies anterior to the IVC and SMA, and posterior to the proper hepatic artery and the common bile duct (CBD).
- The portal vein is only a few centimeters in length and approximately 1 cm in diameter.
- The portal vein, proper hepatic artery and CBD enter the liver at the porta hepatis as the 'portal triad.'
- The portal vein divides into right and left branches at the porta hepatis to accompany hepatic artery and bile duct branches into the liver.
- The portal veins divide the liver into superior and inferior segments.
- The left portal vein is accompanied by the ligamentum teres and the ligamentum venosum.

Hepatic veins (Fig. 9.1)

- Three main hepatic veins pass from the back of the liver to the IVC immediately below the diaphragm.
- The most common pattern is a right hepatic vein that drains independently and a common trunk for the middle and left hepatic veins (two-thirds of individuals).
- The hepatic veins divide the liver into anterior and posterior segments.
- A less common pattern is for the three hepatic veins to drain independently into the IVC.

Liver

- Of the blood supply to the liver, 75–80% is from the portal vein. Blood from the bowel, spleen and viscera is partially deoxygenated.
- Of the blood supply to the liver, 20–25% is from the hepatic artery. Blood from the systemic system is oxygenated.
- There are eight segments of the liver (Fig. 9.2) based on the vascular system as described by Couinaud.*
- Each segment has a portal vein branch in the centre and a hepatic vein at its margin.
- The middle hepatic vein divides the right and left lobes.

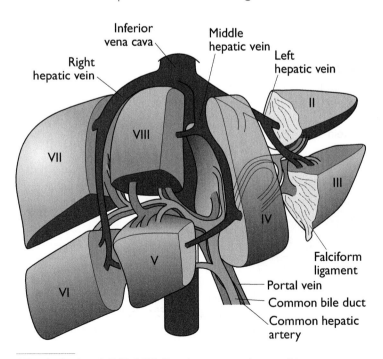

Fig. 9.2 *Normal segmental anatomy of the liver.*

---

*Claude Couinaud, 1922–2008, French surgeon and anatomist

Right lobe
- It is the largest lobe and lies to the right of the midline.
- It is supplied by the right portal vein.
- It is divided by the right hepatic vein into anterior (V and VIII) and posterior (VI and VII) segments.
- It lies anterior to the right kidney.

Left lobe
- It lies in the epigastrium, in part to the left and the rest to the right of the midline.
- It lies anterior to the aorta.
- It is supplied by the left portal vein.
- The ligamentum teres is a remnant of the fetal umbilical vein and lies in the free edge of the falciform ligament of the liver or can extend superficially from the anterior aspect of the left portal vein.
- The ligamentum teres can recanalize to re-form the paraumbilical vein.
- The ligamentum teres and left hepatic vein divide the left lobe into medial (quadrate; IVa and IVb) and lateral (II and III) segments.
- Segment IVb lies adjacent to the gallbladder.

Caudate lobe
- It is smaller than the right and left lobes.
- It forms segment I.
- It is supplied by branches of both left and right portal veins.
- It is drained by emissary hepatic veins straight into the IVC.
- It is situated on the posterosuperior surface of the liver on the right lobe of liver opposite the thoracic vertebrae T10 and T11.
- It is bounded on the left side by the ligamentum teres, below by the porta hepatis, and on the right by the fossa for the IVC.

Portosystemic collaterals (Fig. 9.3)
- There are several potential sites for anastomosis between portal and systemic venous tributaries.

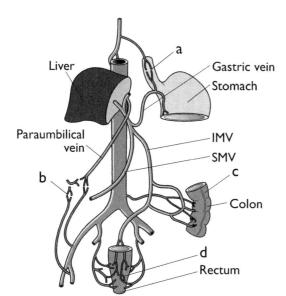

Fig. 9.3 *Potential sites for anastomosis between intra-abdominal portal and systemic venous collaterals:*
a Esophagus.
b Umbilicus.
c Colon.
d Rectum.

- These can lead to varices if hepatoportal drainage is compromised, and can rupture causing hemorrhage.
- Coronary vein tributaries connect to systemic esophageal veins, potentially resulting in varices at the gastroesophageal junction (Fig. 9.3a).
- The paraumbilical vein joins the left branch of the portal vein through the ligamentum teres to connect with systemic veins of the abdominal wall at the umbilicus (Fig. 9.3b).
- IMV tributaries connect with veins draining to the internal iliac veins at the colon and rectum (Fig. 9.3c,d).
- Splenosystemic collaterals pass to the pancreatic head or gastroesophageal region.
- Splenorenal collaterals connect the splenic vein with the left renal vein, usually at the hilum of the spleen.
- Retroperitoneal varices can form a 'tumor-like' mass.

Anatomical variations
Portal veins
- Portal vein trifurcation.
- Right anterior portal branch arising from the left portal vein.
- Right posterior portal branch arising from the main portal vein.
- Agenesis of the right or left portal vein.

Hepatic veins
- Small right hepatic vein compensated by a large right inferior hepatic vein, an accessory vein or well-developed middle hepatic vein.
- A fourth hepatic vein from the left or middle hepatic vein or IVC.

Liver
- Riedel's lobe can be seen extending inferior from the right lobe, lying anterior to the right kidney.
- Lack of development of segments II and III of the left lobe leading to compensatory hypertrophy of the right lobe and quadrate segment of the left lobe.

CLINICAL ASPECTS
Regional pathology
Prehepatic venous thrombosis
- Portal or splenic vein thrombosis usually results from portal hypertension due to cirrhosis.
- Of patients with cirrhosis, 5–20% will develop portal vein thrombosis.
- Thrombosis can also result from coagulation disorders, malignancy, intra-abdominal sepsis or unknown causes.
- Extrinsic portal vein obstruction can result from pancreatitis, pancreatic carcinoma or hepatocellular carcinoma.
- SMV thrombosis alone is less common.
- Splenic vein thrombosis alone leads to less severe clinical sequela due to a more extensive collateral network.
- Thrombosis may be partially or fully occlusive.
- Thrombosis may affect only one branch.
- In the late phase, a thrombosed portal vein becomes small and is replaced by collaterals or a cavernous venous malformation at the porta hepatis.

Intrahepatic disease
- Alcoholic cirrhosis.
- Posthepatitis cirrhosis.
- Idiopathic non-cirrhotic portal fibrosis.
- Cirrhosis may later be complicated by hepatocellular carcinoma.

Posthepatic venous thrombosis (Budd–Chiari syndrome)
- There are several possible causes:
  - Hepatic venous or suprahepatic IVC thrombosis commonly associated with myeloproliferative disorders or thrombophilia.
  - Extrinsic hepatic vein compression by hepatic tumors.
  - Extrinsic hepatic vein compression by a large caudate lobe.
  - Congenital IVC web mostly in Asian individuals.
  - Oral contraceptive pill.
- It is classified as primary when caused by thrombosis or a congenital web and secondary when due to extrinsic compression.
- The syndrome consists of hepatosplenomegaly, ascites and upper abdominal pain.
- Not all hepatic veins are necessarily involved.
- There is congestive liver damage, the severity of which is determined by the extent of thrombosis and the development of venous collaterals.

Portal hypertension
- Portal hypertension results from pre-, intra- or posthepatic causes.
- There is elevated pressure in the portal venous system due to increased resistance to flow resulting in splanchnic vasodilation.
- Flow is diverted to lower-pressure systemic veins through collaterals to shunt blood away from the portal system.
- Variceal collaterals are thin-walled and prone to rupture under high pressure causing gastrointestinal bleeding.

Clinical presentations
- The severity of symptoms depends on the extent and location of thrombus and the degree of collateral development.
- Presentations of a failing liver transplant are similar.

Gastrointestinal hemorrhage
- Hemorrhage can result from increased pressure in portosystemic collaterals, particularly from submucosal varices in the lower esophagus or cardia and fundus of the stomach.
- This occurs in some 50% of patients with cirrhosis and has an immediate mortality rate of >10%.
- There is an approximate 50% risk of rebleeding and a 50% mortality rate within 1–2 years without treatment.
- The incidence of hemorrhage is high if flow in collaterals is towards the superior vena cava (SVC) and low if flow is towards the IVC.
- There is splenomegaly and anemia due to hypersplenism in approximately 50%.

Ascites
- Ascites is most often secondary to chronic liver disease rather than acute liver failure.

- It is usually a relatively early presentation and may be precipitated by fluid retention, heart failure or intraperitoneal malignancy.

Hepatic encephalopathy
- Shunting blood flow from the portal to systemic circulation through either collaterals or a surgical connection can cause a toxic neurological deficit.
- The liver normally detoxifies products from the digestive tract, and portosystemic shunting diverts these toxic products into the systemic circulation.
- Breakdown products of protein metabolism are particularly toxic.
- Spontaneous development has an insidious onset with intellectual deterioration, whereas advanced stages can lead to coma.

Hepatorenal syndrome
- This is a severe complication of advanced liver disease with portal hypertension and ascites.
- It can be precipitated by shock, infection, surgery, large-volume paracentesis or nephrotoxic drugs.
- It results from intense splanchnic vasodilation causing reduced effective blood volume and leading to renal vasoconstriction and rapid deterioration of renal function.
- The process is reversible with treatment.

Endocrine dysfunction
- Hypothyroidism, and feminization and hypogonadism in males, are features of liver disease due to failure to metabolize pituitary hormones.

Coagulation disorders
- Increased risk of bleeding in liver disease results from failure to synthesize coagulation factors.

Treatment
Medical treatment
- Control of diet to reduce production of toxic metabolites.
- Various medications of uncertain value.

Surgical portosystemic shunting
- This has been the traditional technique for decompressing the portal venous circulation.
- The object is to prevent recurrence of hemorrhage from varices.
- However, it is a major operation with appreciable mortality; it can cause hepatic encephalopathy and interferes with the ability to use vessels to anastomose for liver transplantation.
- Various techniques are available (Fig. 9.4).
- Anastomosis of the portal vein to the IVC is a non-selective shunt and diverts all portal venous flow from the liver.
- Anastomosis of the splenic vein to the left renal vein is a selective shunt that preserves portal venous flow to the liver.

Percutaneous transjugular intrahepatic portosystemic shunting (TIPS)
- This has largely replaced surgical shunting, with percutaneous insertion via the internal jugular vein of a stent between the intrahepatic branches of the portal vein and a hepatic vein (Fig. 9.5).

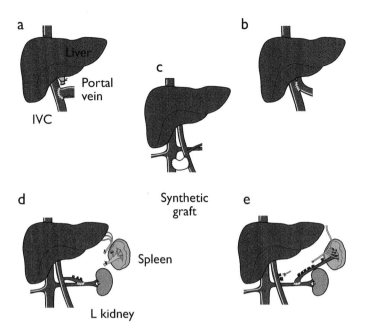

Fig. 9.4 *Portosystemic surgical shunts. a–c are non-selective shunts; d, e are splenorenal shunts.*

a *End-to-side anastomosis portal vein to IVC to divert all portal blood into the systemic circulation.*

b *Side-to-side anastomosis portal vein to IVC to divert some flow but partially preserve portal flow to the liver.*

c *Synthetic bypass from portal vein to IVC if the veins cannot be brought together.*

d *End-to-side anastomosis of proximal splenic vein to left renal vein in order to preserve the portal vein.*

e *End-to-side anastomosis distal splenic vein to left renal vein.*

Redrawn from Fig. 101-4, Terblanche J. In: Rutherford RB (ed.), Vascular Surgery. Philadelphia: WB Saunders, 1995. Reproduced with permission.

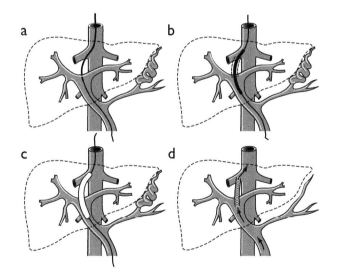

Fig. 9.5 *The technique for TIPS:*

a *Percutaneous puncture to thread a needle-tipped guidewire through the internal jugular vein to the IVC and through a hepatic vein to a portal vein branch.*

b *A balloon threaded over the wire is expanded to form a track between the two circulations and is then removed.*

c *A stent is then threaded over the wire and deployed in the track.*

d *The deployed stent maintains a channel between the two circulations.*

Redrawn from Fig. 101-3, Terblanche J. In: Rutherford RB (ed.), Vascular Surgery. Philadelphia: WB Saunders, 1995. Reproduced with permission.

- TIPS is equivalent to side-to-side portocaval shunting.
- It does not interfere with the subsequent ability to perform liver transplantation.
- It can be complicated by hepatic encephalopathy, thrombosis, hemorrhage or the need to repeat the procedure.

- TIPS may be the definitive treatment for portal hypertension but it has a high restenosis rate.
- Alternately, TIPS may be used as a temporary measure while awaiting liver transplantation.
- The procedure is usually performed under fluoroscopic control.
- Liver function may improve and hepatic hemodynamics may return towards normal after TIPS due to hypertrophy of remaining non-cirrhotic liver tissue.

Liver transplantation

- Transplantation has become widely accepted as the definitive treatment for advanced liver disease as immunosuppression techniques have become more effective.
- It may be required for liver failure from cirrhosis due to hepatitis C, alcohol-related cirrhosis, portal or hepatic vein thrombosis, biliary atresia, refractory ascites, the hepatorenal syndrome or malignancy.
- Typically, the donor liver is removed with a length of CBD, portal vein, hepatic artery and IVC, and replaces the diseased liver with anastomosis of each. There are several variations of this technique (Fig. 9.6).

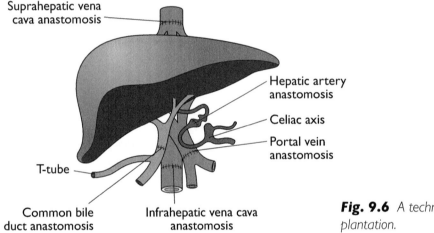

Fig. 9.6 *A technique for liver transplantation.*

Selection of treatment

- Primary bleeding is not usually an indication for prophylaxis by surgical intervention.
- Active bleeding can be controlled by balloon tamponade and pharmacological agents that cause venoconstriction.
- Endoscopic techniques are then used to sclerose or ligate varices.

Indications for shunting or TIPS

- Intractable variceal hemorrhage.
- Recurrent variceal bleeding after failure of endoscopic treatment.
- Refractory ascites.
- Budd–Chiari syndrome and veno-occlusive disease.

Contraindications to shunting or TIPS

- Progressive liver failure, pulmonary hypertension or severe hepatic encephalopathy.
- Thrombosis in veins to be considered for shunting.

Indications for liver transplantation

- End-stage acute liver failure.
- Advanced cirrhosis.
- Congenital metabolic disorders with inadequate liver function.
- Primary hepatic carcinoma confined to the liver usually after reduction in tumor size by preliminary local chemotherapy and embolization.

Complications
Surgical portosystemic shunting

- Anastomotic stenosis.

TIPS

- Stenosis or occlusion of stent.

Liver transplantation

- A complication is stenosis or thrombosis of the anastomosed hepatic artery, portal vein or IVC.
- Hepatic artery thrombosis is most common in the first 6 weeks post-transplantation.
- The allograft may be preserved via collaterals when the hepatic artery is fully thrombosed.
- Any increase in portal venous or hepatic arterial flow velocities at the anastomosis sites is likely to lead to further investigation.
- Stenoses may be resolved with percutaneous transhepatic dilation. Failing this, revision of the anastomosis site or portosystemic shunting may save a failing allograft.
- Stenosis or occlusion of the IVC is rare but is usually due to compression by a fluid collection or surgical problems.
- Another complication is liver infarction.
- A false aneurysm may be caused by infection or defective vascular reconstruction and most commonly occurs at the hepatic artery anastomosis site.
- A false aneurysm is often asymptomatic and has the potential to rupture.
- Obstructed draining bile ducts with bile leakage is a common complication.
- Bile leakage is difficult to distinguish from other fluid collections such as ascites or hematoma.
- Acute allograft rejection is the most common serious complication. Treatment is usually adjustment of the immunosuppressive drug therapy and is usually successful.
- Ultrasound is an important modality for long-term follow-up of liver transplants.

WHAT DOCTORS NEED TO KNOW

- Is there thrombosis or occlusion of the portal vein, its tributaries, the hepatic veins or IVC?
- Are the veins to be considered for portosystemic shunting patent?
- Are collateral veins and portosystemic venous connections present?
- Are venous connections or vascular anastomoses patent or stenosed after portosystemic shunting, TIPS or liver transplantation and what are their sizes?
- What is the diameter of the CBD?
- What are the sizes of the liver and spleen?
- What is the composition of the liver?
- Is ascites present?

THE DUPLEX SCAN

Abbreviation

- Resistance index – RI = (peak systolic velocity – end-diastolic velocity)/peak systolic velocity

Indications for scanning

Clinical indications

- Abdominal pain.
- Ascites.
- Hepatosplenomegaly.
- Symptoms of liver failure.
- Gastrointestinal bleeding.
- Pancreatic disease.

Selection for intervention

- Examine for normal anatomy of the portal veins, hepatic veins, IVC, hepatic artery and biliary system.
- Note hepatic tumors or other diseases.
- If there is any uncertainty then investigation is likely to proceed to angiography or other imaging techniques.

Surveillance after intervention

- The very high incidence of stent stenosis or occlusion in the stent after TIPS makes postoperative surveillance essential.
- Scanning is recommended at 48 hours to 1 week post-TIPS, every 3 months for the first year and then 6-monthly.

Normal findings

Portal and hepatic venous flow

- Normal portal venous flow is always towards the liver (*hepatopetal*). Flow in the hepatic artery and branches is in the same direction and it can be difficult to distinguish between them with color Doppler.
- The portal venous waveform shows continuous flow with average velocity 15–20 cm/s which is not pulsatile but is phasic with respiration such that flow tends to fall during inspiration and rise during expiration (Fig. 9.7).
- Portal venous flow characteristics change with posture and after exercise or a meal.
- All vein lumina should be smooth and anechoic on B-mode and should fill with color Doppler.
- The portal vein diameter measured where it crosses the IVC is <13 mm with quiet respiration increasing to <16 mm with deep inspiration.
- SMV and splenic vein diameters increase by 20–100% during inspiration and decrease with expiration.
- Portal vein and SMV flow and diameters increase after a meal whereas flow falls after exercise.
- Hepatic veins show triphasic flow reflecting the right heart signal as well as respiratory fluctuations (Fig. 9.8).
- It should be possible to identify three patent hepatic veins.

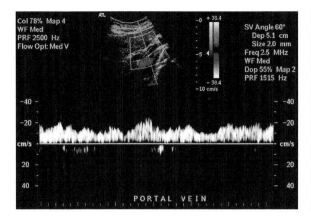

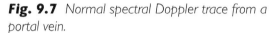

Fig. 9.7 *Normal spectral Doppler trace from a portal vein.*

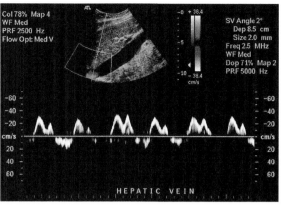

Fig. 9.8 *Normal spectral Doppler trace from a hepatic vein.*

Liver, spleen, and CBD
- Smooth liver surface.
- Homogeneous liver echogenicity; same or brighter echogenicity than adjacent right renal cortex.
- Liver length <15.5 cm.
- Spleen length <13 cm.
- CBD diameter <5 mm, with a normal increase in diameter by 1 mm for each decade over age 50 years.
- First-order intrahepatic bile duct diameter approximately 2 mm.

Hepatic artery flow
- RI is the most common Doppler ultrasound parameter used to evaluate hepatic artery flow.
- The usual range in normal as well as post-transplant recipients is 0.55–0.80.

Normal findings after intervention
Surgical portosystemic shunting
- Surgical shunts may be difficult to visualize with ultrasound.
- Indirect evidence of shunt patency is useful.
- Flow through the anastomosis from the portal to systemic circulation is shown by color and spectral Doppler.
- There is dilation of the IVC or other recipient vein.
- There is a reduction in size and number of collaterals.
- There is phasic flow with respiration in portal vein tributaries.
- Flow away from the liver (*hepatofugal*) in intrahepatic portal veins occurs if a side-to-side portocaval shunt has been performed.
- Hepatofugal flow in the splenic vein occurs after splenorenal shunting with a large left renal vein directing flow to the IVC.
- There is reduced ascites and splenomegaly.

TIPS

- Hepatopetal flow in the splenic and main portal vein although there may be hepatofugal flow in intrahepatic portal veins.
- Maximum portal venous velocity double normal values to 30-40 cm/s with spectral broadening from turbulence and respiratory and cardiac fluctuations of flow.
- Velocities in the stent ranging from 90 cm/s to 190cm/s.
- Similar velocities at the portal and hepatic ends of the stent.
- Similar velocities within the stent on serial scans.
- Pulsatile turbulent flow in the stent.
- Portal vein diameter possibly increasing.
- Hepatic artery velocity increasing by >50%.
- Decrease in the number and size of collaterals.
- Reduced ascites and splenomegaly.

Liver transplantation

- Smooth liver surface.
- Homogeneous liver echogenicity.
- Small amount of residual ascites possibly present.
- Normal CBD diameter.
- Patent hepatic artery, portal vein, IVC, and hepatic veins.
- Hepatopetal flow in the portal vein.
- Gradual return of hepatic artery RI to normal.

Criteria for diagnosing disease

Portal hypertension

- Hepatopetal flow with a reduced velocity with minor disease, to-and-fro (biphasic) portal venous flow with moderate disease (Fig. 9.9), and hepatofugal portal venous flow with severe disease is diagnostic.
- Hepatofugal portal venous flow always indicates disease.
- Increased phasicity in hepatofugal portal venous flow is due to increase in hepatic artery flow compensating for the decrease in portal venous flow.
- The presence of portosystemic collaterals or varices is highly specific (Fig. 9.10).
- Demonstration of a patent paraumbilical vein ≥3 mm diameter with hepatofugal flow in the ligamentum teres is a highly specific and sensitive sign for intra- or posthepatic portal hypertension (Fig. 9.11).
- Hepatopetal flow may be seen in the main and left portal vein leading to the recanalized paraumbilical vein with hepatofugal flow in the right portal vein (Fig. 9.12).
- Enlarged portal vein >13 mm with quiet respiration in a fasting patient lying supine is present in approximately 50% and is highly specific.
- Enlarged left gastric vein and coronary vein are >6–7 mm diameter.
- Decreased portal vein flow velocity is highly variable.
- Change of the cross-sectional shape of the portal vein is from elliptical to circular.
- Less than a 20% increase in splenic vein or SMV diameter, with change from quiet respiration to deep inspiration is specific and sensitive but difficult in practice.
- Thready hepatic veins are difficult to sample.
- There is the presence of abnormal liver texture.
- Splenomegaly (length >13 cm) is present in 50%.
- There is ascites (Fig. 9.11).

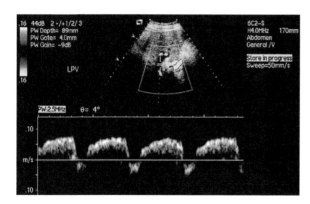

Fig. 9.9 *Spectral Doppler trace demonstrating biphasic flow in the portal vein due to portal hypertension.*

Image kindly supplied by Martin Necas, Hamilton, New Zealand.

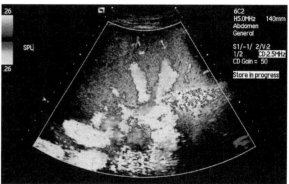

Fig. 9.10 *Color Doppler demonstrating large splenosystemic varices.*

Image kindly supplied by Martin Necas, Hamilton, New Zealand.

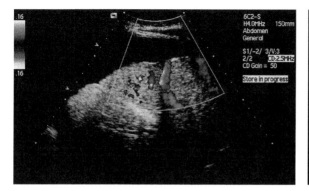

Fig. 9.11 *Color Doppler demonstrating a recanalized paraumbilical vein.*
- *Note ascites shown as an echolucent area.*

Image kindly supplied by Martin Necas, Hamilton, New Zealand.

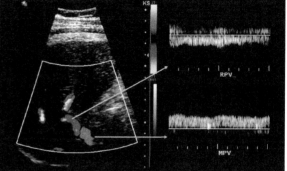

Fig. 9.12 *Spectral Doppler demonstrating flow directions in the right and middle portal veins due to portal hypertension and a recanalized paraumbilical vein.*

Image kindly supplied by Martin Necas, Hamilton, New Zealand.

Portal vein thrombosis

- Enlarged portal vein filled with echogenic material if acute (Fig. 9.13).
- Small, echogenic portal vein if there is chronic occlusion.
- No evidence of venous flow in the portal vein or at the porta hepatis when Doppler sensitivity has been maximized.
- Cavernous transformation of the portal vein with tortuous collaterals at the porta hepatis – these demonstrate the same flow pattern as the now thrombosed portal vein (Fig. 9.14).
- Loss of diameter fluctuations with respiration.
- Numerous large varices representing portosystemic shunts with continuous low-velocity portal venous flow.
- A coronary vein diameter >6–7 mm.
- Increased and more pulsatile hepatic arterial flow with arterial dilation. RI >0.8.

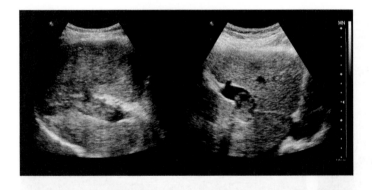

Fig. 9.13 *B-mode image of portal vein thrombosis.*

Image kindly supplied by Martin Necas, Hamilton, New Zealand.

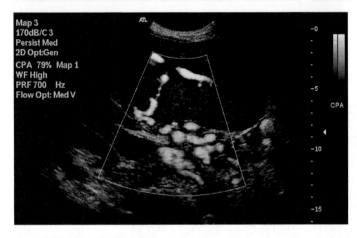

Fig. 9.14 *Power Doppler of cavernous transformation of the portal vein.*

Image kindly supplied by Martin Necas, Hamilton, New Zealand.

Budd–Chiari syndrome

- Hepatic veins:
  - No color or spectral flow signal if thrombosed.
  - Reversed, turbulent, monophasic, or biphasic flow if patent.
  - Loss of phasicity suggesting IVC occlusion.
  - Thickened vein wall and vein dilation.
  - Intrahepatic collaterals.
  - Abnormal vein course.
  - Extrahepatic anastomoses.
- IVC:
  - Abnormal, reversed, or absent flow.
  - Thrombosis, stenosis, or membrane.

Portosystemic collaterals

- Ultrasound underestimates the extent of the collateral network.
- The coronary vein can be difficult to identify because its origin and course are variable, particularly if the patient is obese.
- Flow reduction in the portal vein, with reversed flow in the splenic vein, suggests splenorenal collaterals.
- Reversed flow in the SMV may indicate collaterals between the mesenteric veins and systemic circulation.

Esophageal varices

- If hepatofugal flow in the paraumbilical vein exceeds hepatopetal flow in the portal vein then bleeding from esophageal varices is extremely unlikely.
- If hepatopetal flow in the portal vein exceeds hepatofugal flow through the paraumbilical vein then esophageal variceal bleeding is likely.

Liver disease

- B-mode can be used to distinguish diffuse liver disease due to cirrhosis (nodular liver surface and heterogeneous texture with increased reflectivity), non-cirrhotic portal fibrosis (diffuse texture) or fatty infiltration (increased parenchymal echogenicity) with moderate accuracy.
- B-mode also detects liver tumors and color Doppler is used to assess their vascularity.
- Triphasic flow becomes biphasic or monophasic in hepatic veins with more severe cirrhosis, due to reduced elasticity of the liver (Fig. 9.15).
- Hepatomegaly occurs with acute cirrhosis; liver length >15.5 cm.
- Hepatomegaly can also be diagnosed by enlargement of the caudate lobe in comparison to the right lobe. A ratio of >0.65 is diagnostic.
- The liver atrophies with chronic cirrhosis.
- An indication of hepatomegaly is the loss of the sharp edge at the deep surface of the liver to a rounded shape.
- Ultrasound provides additional information about liver, biliary, splenic or pancreatic disease.
- Splanchnic hemodynamics differ for chronic liver diseases and hematological diseases causing splenomegaly.
- Splenomegaly due to cirrhosis causes decreased portal flow velocity, increased splenic artery resistance and large esophageal varices whereas these findings are not observed with primary splenomegaly.

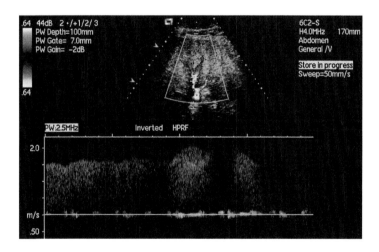

Fig. 9.15 *Spectral Doppler trace of monophasic high-velocity flow with spectral broadening in a hepatic vein.*
Image kindly supplied by Martin Necas, Hamilton, New Zealand.

Criteria for diagnosing disease after intervention
Surgical portosystemic shunt stenosis

- Stenosis at the anastomosis after shunting or transplantation will result in reversion to features of portal hypertension.
- Criteria that indicate anastomotic stenosis have not been defined.
- Any increase above the normal maximum flow velocity of 40 cm/s is likely to lead to further investigation.

TIPS stenosis and occlusion

- The most common site for stenosis is at the junction of the stent and the hepatic vein.
- Stent stenosis will cause the maximum velocity to fall to <90–100 cm/s in the portal vein and rise to >190–200 cm/s with post-stenotic turbulence in the stent.
- There is a change in velocity >100 cm/s across the stent.
- There is visible narrowing with color Doppler.
- Stent occlusion results in absent flow with color and spectral Doppler within the stent and to either side.
- There is hepatofugal or to-and-fro flow in the main portal or splenic veins.
- There is an increase in stent velocity >50 cm/s on serial scan.
- There is a recurrence of portosystemic variceal bleeding.
- There is development of splenomegaly and ascites.

Liver transplantation complications

- There can be stenosis or thrombosis of the anastomosed hepatic artery, portal vein or IVC.
- Hepatic artery thrombosis is most common in the first 6 weeks post-transplantation.
- Thrombosis is confirmed by lack of flow with color and spectral Doppler. There may be collateral vessel formation.
- Intrahepatic waveforms may remain normal even with full hepatic artery thrombosis due to collateral supply.
- Criteria that indicate anastomotic stenosis have not been defined.
- Any increase in portal venous or hepatic arterial flow velocities at the anastomoses is likely to lead to further investigation.
- Severe hepatic artery stenosis leads to an intrahepatic 'tardus parvus' waveform (see Chapter 7, page 133) on spectral Doppler.
- Signs of portal vein stenosis include post-stenotic dilation and the formation of collaterals.
- Increase of the peak velocity to >100 cm/s or fourfold increase in velocity at the site of narrowing indicates a portal vein stenosis.
- Turbulence in the portal vein does not necessarily indicate stenosis due to some infolding at the anastomosis site.
- Visualization of narrowing and post-stenotic dilation on B-mode with increased velocities and turbulent flow with color and spectral Doppler, indicates hepatic vein or IVC stenosis.
- Liver infarction is demonstrated with B-mode as areas of heterogeneity and decreased echogenicity.
- A false aneurysm is shown with color Doppler as a localized outpouching with turbulent arterial flow.
- Dilation of intrahepatic bile ducts is more useful in demonstrating obstructed bile ducts than the diameter of the CBD. Increase in diameters of these bile ducts on serial ultrasounds indicates obstruction.
- Bile leakage is demonstrated as echolucent fluid collection near the CBD anastomosis site.
- Unlike kidney transplants with increased renal artery RI, rejection of liver transplants is not associated with increased hepatic artery RI.

PROTOCOLS FOR SCANNING

- Preparing the patient, selecting the best transducer, and general principles for scanning are discussed in Chapter 3 (pages 40–42).
- The patient may need prior abdominal paracentesis if there is marked ascites.

Position the patient and select windows

- Lay the patient supine.
- If the scan is difficult, move to a left lateral decubitus position. The liver is an acoustic window providing clear imaging of the porta hepatis.
- Right lateral decubitus may be suitable to image the splenic vein. Have the patient take in a large breath to displace the spleen down for a better acoustic window.
- Tilt the patient into slight reverse Trendelenberg to allow the viscera to descend if bowel gas is a problem.
- Suitable windows include the following:
  - Right subcostal or intercostal coronal window for the portal veins, hepatic artery and CBD.
  - Left intercostal and subcostal coronal window through the spleen for the distal splenic vein and spleen length.
  - Right subcostal transverse oblique window for the left and middle hepatic and TIPS.
  - Right intercostal window for the right hepatic vein and xiphisternum window for the left and middle hepatic veins.
  - Right intercostal transverse window for the right hepatic vein or TIPS stent.

How to differentiate portal and hepatic veins in the liver

- Both are seen as echolucent structures.
- The portal triad is surrounded by a dense fibrous sheath.
- Hepatic veins are larger than portal veins and do not have valves.
- Portal veins are larger at the porta hepatis and hepatic veins enlarge as they pass towards the IVC.
- Portal veins converge at the porta hepatis and hepatic veins converge as they pass towards the IVC.
- Portal veins tend to run transversely and hepatic veins to run longitudinally.
- Portal venous flow is phasic with respiration whereas hepatic venous flow is phasic but also reflects right atrial pulsations.

Scan the extra and intrahepatic portal veins, SMV, splenic vein and hepatic artery

- Set color and spectral Doppler sensitivity to recognize low-flow states.
- Examine the veins in B-mode and color Doppler.
- Take sample spectral traces to determine patency, flow direction and waveform morphology.
- Measure diameters in B-mode for each vein. Measure the portal vein diameter where it crosses anterior to the IVC.
- Identify the splenic vein near the midline; follow it to the left as it passes transverse then deeper and cephalad to the hilum of the spleen. It may be impossible to visualize the full length of the splenic vein.
- Trace the splenic vein to the right to its junction with the portal vein to distinguish the portal vein from the IVC and bile ducts.
- Follow the portal vein cephalad to its division into right and left portal veins near the porta hepatis.
- With color Doppler examine for cavernous transformation of the portal vein at the portal hepatis.
- Using color and spectral Doppler, examine for flow in the posterior and anterior branches of the right portal vein. Posterior branch flow will be away from the transducer.

- Then follow the portal vein caudally and medially to its origin.
- View the SMV in longitudinal from its confluence with the splenic vein and in spectral Doppler take spectral traces to distinguish it from the SMA.
- At the porta hepatis, identify the hepatic artery and with spectral Doppler determine the hepatic artery RI.

CBD

- In B-mode and longitudinal, measure the diameter of the CBD at the porta hepatis as it crosses anterior to the hepatic artery.

Ascites

- Identify the presence of ascites.
- On B-mode, ascites appears echolucent.
- The echolucent areas can surround the liver and bowel loops.

Scan the liver

- In B-mode, examine the liver surface and texture.
- Remember to switch to a high-frequency linear transducer when scanning the liver surface.
- The best image for examining the surface is of the anterior border of the left lobe because it cannot be compressed by the chest wall.
- All liver segments must be scanned in both longitudinal and transverse planes for a thorough evaluation of the parenchyma. Scan beyond the liver capsule.
- In B-mode, measure the craniocaudal length of the right lobe at the right midclavicular line.
- In B-mode, measure the craniocaudal length of the caudate lobe at the right midclavicular line. Calculate caudate:right lobe ratio.

Scan the spleen

- No consensus as to accepted method for measuring spleen size.
- Best measured on the axillary line.
- In B-mode, manipulate the transducer until the maximum craniocaudal length of the spleen is identified.
- Record the length of the spleen.

Scan hepatic veins and IVC

- Examine the veins in B-mode and color and spectral Doppler.
- Take sample spectral traces to determine patency, flow direction and waveform morphology.
- Use color and spectral Doppler to demonstrate partial or lack of flow due to thrombus.
- Use B-mode to measure diameters for each vein.
- Use B-mode to demonstrate venous webs in the IVC.
- Scan more cephalad to examine each hepatic vein as it passes to the IVC near the right atrium.
- Use color Doppler because the veins can be difficult to identify with B-mode alone particularly if there is extrinsic compression.

TIP!

- The Valsalva maneuver may elicit hepatofugal flow if there is difficulty obtaining spectral traces in low-flow veins.

Scan portosystemic collateral veins

- Identify tortuous collaterals in B-mode and color Doppler.
- Take sample spectral traces to indicate their presence and flow direction.
- In B-mode, measure the anteroposterior diameters of varices and the paraumbilical vein.
- Scan in longitudinal for the coronary vein extending cephalad from the SMV near its confluence with the portal vein.
- Scan for the paraumbilical vein in the ligamentum teres in transverse and longitudinal. In B-mode, it is identified as a hypoechoic channel within the echogenic band of the ligamentum teres. Alternately, scan from the umbilicus on the anterior abdominal wall and follow more cephalad.
- With color and spectral Doppler, determine patency and direction of flow of the paraumbilical and coronary veins.

Scan a surgical portosystemic shunt

- Ascertain location of shunt from referral or patient's notes.
- Perform a full hepatoportal venous and hepatic arterial study as described above.
- Take sample spectral traces. Note patency, flow direction and waveform morphology. Record maximum velocities at shunt site or within graft anastomosis sites and the graft.
- It may not be possible to see a distal splenorenal shunt due to overlying bowel gas. However, normal flow in the perihilar segment of the splenic vein indicates shunt patency.

Scan after TIPS

- The stent is easily seen in the liver as a highly echogenic but non-shadowing structure.
- It usually connects a hepatic vein deep in the right lobe and a branch of the portal vein at the porta hepatis.
- With color and spectral Doppler, note patency. Take sample spectral traces to demonstrate velocity, flow direction and waveform morphology in these veins:
  - Portal venous end, midpoint and hepatic venous end of TIPS.
  - Other intrahepatic veins if the stent cannot be clearly seen due to bowel gas.
  - Right and left portal veins.
  - Extrahepatic portal vein.
  - SMV and splenic vein at their confluence.
  - All main hepatic veins.
  - IVC.
- Identify the stent in B-mode in longitudinal, oblique and transverse.
- Note its location and extension into the hepatic and portal veins to detect stent migration with serial scans.

Scan a liver transplant
- Perform the scanning protocols as for the extra- and intrahepatic portal veins, SMV, splenic vein and hepatic artery.
- Pay particular attention to anastomosis sites for stenosis. Take sample spectral traces within anastomosis sites. Record velocities.
- In B-mode, scan for bile leakage.
- Perform the scanning protocol as for the liver.
- In B-mode, measure the diameters of the common, left, and right bile ducts as comparative baseline for further serial ultrasound scans.

ULTRASOUND IMAGES TO RECORD

Portal hypertension
- Sample spectral traces to record flow direction in all vessels.
- Spectral traces of the hepatic arteries at any sites of stenosis or occlusion, noting the extent and location from the vessel origin.
- Record hepatic artery RI.
- Color Doppler to show presence of collaterals and spectral Doppler to show flow directions.
- B-mode for diameters of hepatoportal veins and CBD.
- Color Doppler and spectral traces to show thrombosis of portal or hepatic veins.
- B-mode measurements of the size of the liver and spleen. Note the texture of the liver.
- Perform other pathology such as ascites, hepatic cyst or tumor.

TIPS surveillance
- Sample spectral traces and note velocities, direction of flow and waveform morphology:
  - Portal venous end, midpoint and hepatic venous end of TIPS.
  - Other intrahepatic veins if the stent cannot be clearly seen due to bowel gas.
  - Right and left portal veins.
  - Extrahepatic portal vein.
  - SMV and splenic vein at their confluence.
  - All main hepatic veins.
  - IVC.
- Spectral traces proximal to, at and distal to stent stenosis. Record velocities.
- Spectral traces demonstrating stent occlusion.

Liver transplantation
- Images as for portal hypertension.
- Sample spectral traces within anastomosis sites.
- Spectral traces proximal to, at and distal to stenosis.

WORKSHEET

● Draw a diagram recording waveform morphology and direction of flow in all vessels, presence of collaterals, liver and spleen sizes, liver echotexture and all other relevant ultrasound findings.

VENOUS THROMBOSIS IN THE LOWER LIMBS

10

Ultrasound is the investigation most often used to determine the presence, site and extent of thrombus in deep or superficial veins. The D-dimer pathology test has a high negative predictive value and can be used for screening. Occasionally, patients require computed tomographic venography (CTV) to demonstrate iliac or inferior vena caval thrombosis. Most departments have abandoned other indirect investigations.

ANATOMY

Veins and junctions scanned for reporting – all patients:
- Common femoral vein – CFV
- Profunda femoris vein – PFV
- Femoral vein – FV (previously superficial femoral vein)
- Popliteal vein
- Posterior tibial veins – PTV
- Peroneal veins
- Great saphenous vein – GSV (previously greater, long, internal)
- Small saphenous vein – SSV (previously lesser, short, external)
- Gastrocnemius veins and soleal sinuses
- Saphenofemoral junction – SFJ
- Saphenopopliteal junction – SPJ.

Veins scanned for reporting – selected patients:
- Inferior vena cava – IVC
- Common iliac vein – CIV
- Internal iliac vein – IIV
- External iliac vein – EIV
- Anterior tibial veins – ATV.

- The anatomy of deep veins is discussed in this chapter
- The anatomy of superficial veins is discussed in Chapter 11 as are the changes in terminology.

IVC, iliac and gonadal veins (Fig. 10.1)
- The IVC is to the right of the aorta.
- Each CIV is to the right of the corresponding artery.
- The left CIV is crossed by the right common iliac artery.
- The left gonadal (ovarian or testicular) vein passes vertically upwards to join the left renal vein, which crosses superficial to the aorta and deep to the superior mesenteric artery. It may be duplicated.
- The right gonadal (ovarian or testicular) vein joins the IVC at an anterior oblique upwards direction.
- An anomalous left-sided IVC may be present from persistence of the embryological azygos vein (Fig. 10.2).

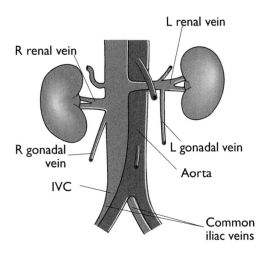

Fig. 10.1 *The infrarenal IVC and common iliac veins.*

Redrawn from Fig. 23.14, Zwiebel WJ. Introduction to Vascular Ultrasonography. Philadelphia: WB Saunders, 1994. Reproduced with permission.

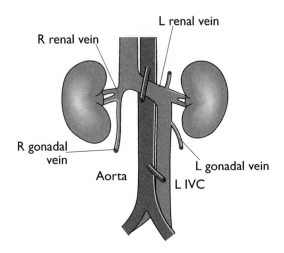

Fig. 10.2 *Anomalous left-sided IVC.*

Redrawn from Fig. 23.14, Zwiebel WJ. Introduction to Vascular Ultrasonography. Philadelphia: WB Saunders, 1994. Reproduced with permission.

Femoral and popliteal veins (Fig. 10.3)
- The veins wind around the corresponding arteries.
- They are larger than the arteries.
- The FV and popliteal veins are duplicated in 10% of limbs.

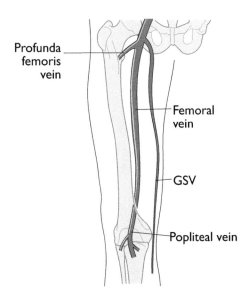

Fig. 10.3 *The femoral and popliteal veins.*

Figure kindly supplied by Trevor Beckwith, Wagga Wagga, Australia, 1996.

Tibial veins, gastrocnemius veins and soleal sinuses (Fig. 10.4)
- The PTV, ATV and peroneal veins follow their corresponding arteries.
- They are usually duplicated.
- The ATV passes through the interosseous membrane.

- The gastrocnemius veins and soleal sinuses are paired and pass to the medial and lateral parts of the corresponding muscles.
- The gastrocnemius veins may join the popliteal vein, upper SSV or confluence at the SPJ.
- The soleal veins join the popliteal vein.

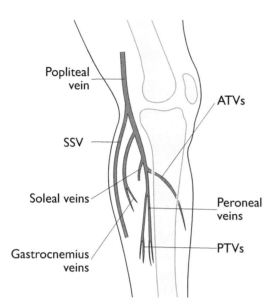

Fig. 10.4 *Tibial veins, gastrocnemius veins and soleal sinuses.*

Figure kindly supplied by Trevor Beckwith, Wagga Wagga, Australia, 1996.

CLINICAL ASPECTS

Pathogenesis
Propagation
- Thrombosis commonly commences in the calf veins particularly at valve sinuses.
- Thrombus can propagate along a vein, initially '*free floating*' and not fixed to the wall subsequently becoming adherent.

Recanalization
- With time, the vein wall produces thrombolytic factors that can recanalize the vein.
- However, this usually causes irreversible damage to venous valves so that venous reflux then occurs under the effect of gravity.
- Some 75% of deep vein thromboses (DVTs) recanalize within 6 months and approximately two-thirds of these develop deep venous reflux.

Occlusion
- If inherent thrombolysis is ineffective, there will be persisting occlusion.
- Whether or not veins remain permanently occluded or reopen is unpredictable and depends in part on the extent of thrombosis and the efficacy of treatment.
- The lumen is filled with thrombus for up to several months.
- Later, the vein may remain filled with a mucoid material but more often it becomes completely sclerosed as a fibrous cord.
- Collateral veins develop to a varying degree.

Clinical presentations

- Venous thrombosis can cause a DVT or superficial thrombophlebitis (STP).
- These can lead to a pulmonary embolism (PE).
- A DVT is considerably more common in the legs than in the arms.
- Pain is often felt at the site of the thrombosis.
- Femoropopliteal DVT may result in calf edema whereas iliac DVT often causes thigh and calf edema.

STP

- The onset is acute and there is considerable surrounding chemical inflammation often incorrectly thought to represent infection.
- The affected vein is painful, red, hot, easily palpable and tender.
- Thrombosis most often involves the GSV, SSV or major tributaries.
- Thrombus propagates through saphenous junctions or perforators to deep veins in approximately 15% of limbs.
- Approximately 10% detach to cause a PE.

DVT

- Many patients are asymptomatic and many symptomatic patients have other conditions.
- Many patients studied for pain or swelling in the leg do not have a DVT but more than 50% of these have another condition that can be diagnosed by ultrasound.
- If a DVT becomes symptomatic, the clinical features include acute pain, swelling, calf tenderness and a moderately raised temperature.
- Most DVTs start in below-knee veins and approximately 10% propagate to above the knee.
- Extensive iliofemoral thrombosis can reduce the circulation sufficient to threaten viability of the leg; this is termed 'phlegmasia cerulea dolens'.
- If a scan is positive for a DVT, then approximately 30% are bilateral. This does not affect immediate treatment but is of value to assess the long-term prognosis for post-thrombotic syndrome.
- If the initial scan clearly excludes a DVT, conversion to a positive scan is extremely unlikely.
- The first presentation may be with a PE or the condition may be unrecognized until post-thrombotic syndrome develops many years later.
- Approximately 50% of patients develop symptoms due to post-thrombotic syndrome within 10 years after a major DVT.

PE

- Thrombus may break away from veins to pass through the right atrium and ventricle to the pulmonary arteries as a PE.
- PE is most likely in the early stages of thrombosis when a clot is less adherent.
- According to the size of the embolus, presentation may be silent and detected only by investigations, symptomatic without compromising the circulation, catastrophic causing cardiac shock or can be fatal.
- Symptoms of PE include deep chest pain, pleuritic pain and dyspnea.
- Approximately 10–20% of lower limbs with DVT develop PE.
- A patent foramen ovale is present in approximately 30% of the population. An embolus may pass through the right to left atrium to the arterial circulation and frequently to the brain causing a stroke. This is termed a 'paradoxical embolism'.

- A PE is diagnosed by pulmonary computed tomography angiography (CTA) which can be supplemented by CT of the iliofemoral veins and ultrasound for venous thrombosis in the lower limbs.
- Approximately one-third of patients with a PE shown by CTA have a normal ultrasound study of the lower limbs.

Differential diagnosis
STP
- Cellulitis.
- Lymphangitis.
- Eczema.

DVT
- Cellulitis.
- Torn calf muscle.
- Ruptured Baker's cyst.
- Subfascial hematoma.
- Ruptured plantaris muscle.
- Prolonged limb dependency.
- Lymphedema.
- Lymphangitis.
- Nerve entrapment.

Treatment
STP
- STP is treated either by a compression bandage and analgesics or by saphenous vein ligation.
- Anticoagulation is not required and antibiotics are inappropriate.
- STP in the GSV extending to the SFJ or floating into the CFV may require urgent surgery to ligate the junction to prevent PE.

DVT
- A patient with a DVT is now usually treated as an outpatient with compression bandaging and anticoagulation using low-molecular-weight heparin injections initially and oral warfarin for 3–6 months.
- The duration for anticoagulation is influenced by whether serial studies show propagation or recanalization.
- If serial studies show that thrombus is propagating in spite of anticoagulation, treatment needs to be reviewed, possibly with insertion of an IVC filter.
- Permanent anticoagulation may be required if there are associated risk factors such as thrombophilia.
- Occasionally, patients with iliofemoral thrombosis are treated by thrombolysis or surgical thrombectomy.
- Thrombolysis for venous thrombosis can be monitored after the procedure using B-mode and color Doppler to confirm that re-established flow is maintained.
- It is frequently necessary after successful lysis to treat underlying stenosis by balloon dilation, stenting or surgery.

PE

- PE is treated by anticoagulation in hospital.
- Recurring PE in spite of adequate anticoagulation are an indication to place an IVC filter.
- Occasionally, patients with severe circulatory impairment require thrombolysis or pulmonary embolectomy.

WHAT DOCTORS NEED TO KNOW

- Is there venous thrombosis?
- Is there thrombus in superficial veins and how close is it to the saphenous junction?
- Is there projection of thrombus into the adjacent deep vein?
- Is there thrombus in deep veins and if so where?
- Is the process unilateral or bilateral?
- Do serial studies show that a DVT is propagating?
- Do serial studies show that the vein is recanalizing or remains occluded?

IMPORTANT!

- This is a very important scan with the onus on the sonographer to be sure before declaring the study to be normal.
- If there is any doubt about the diagnosis, call the supervising doctor to check the findings.
- The sonographer or supervising doctor should ring the referring doctor immediately if a DVT or floating thrombus in a proximal saphenous vein is detected.
- Do not send the patient home before determining the appropriate management.

THE DUPLEX SCAN

- Studies that compare ultrasound scanning with venography show that the sensitivity for ultrasound is >95% for above-knee thrombosis and >85% for below-knee thrombosis for scans where adequate imaging is obtained.

Indications for scanning

- Patients may be referred with symptoms or signs suggesting STP, DVT or PE.
- Asymptomatic patients may be referred if considered to be at high risk due to recent surgery, prolonged bed rest, lower limb trauma or known thrombophilia.
- Patient surveillance: there is no agreement as to how to follow the patient after a DVT has been confirmed. We perform weekly scans until it is confirmed that the thrombus is not propagating as well as a scan for future reference at completion of anticoagulation.
- The approximate yield is as follows:
  - Leg pain or swelling suspected due to DVT – 30%.
  - DVT as a suspected source of PE – 20%.
  - Asymptomatic patients referred to exclude DVT – 15%.

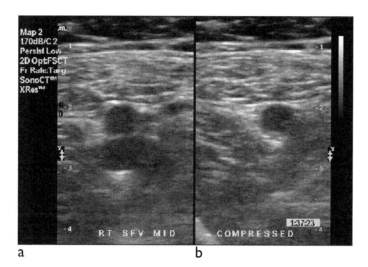

a   b

Fig. 10.5 *B-mode appearance of a normal CFV:*
a *Before compression.*
b *After transducer compression.*

Characteristics of normal veins
- Compressible with transducer pressure (Fig. 10.5).
- Thin walled.
- Larger than the corresponding artery.
- Smooth interior lumen.
- Echo-free lumen.
- Augment with distal compression causing full color filling of the lumen.
- Phasic flow with respiration and cessation of flow with the Valsalva maneuver in upper thigh veins.
- Increase of the CFV diameter by 15–20% with the Valsalva maneuver.

Criteria for diagnosing thrombosis – direct evidence
Inability to compress the vein
- Thrombus prevents the vein walls from coming together with compression.
- The vein can be partially compressed with partially occlusive thrombus but is incompressible with fully occlusive thrombus (Fig. 10.6).

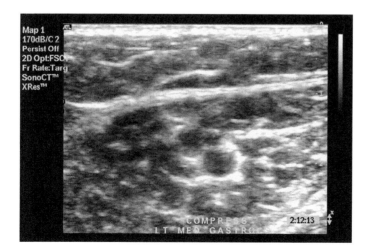

Fig. 10.6 *B-mode appearance incompressible thrombus in medial gastrocnemius veins.*

Intraluminal clot

- Fresh clot is echolucent whereas old thrombus is increasingly echogenic.
- This feature is highly dependent on image quality and instrument settings.

Absent flow in the vein

- There is no flow with occlusive thrombosis and only peripheral flow around a central non-occlusive thrombus (Fig. 10.7).
- This is an important indicator for iliac DVT where it is often not possible to test for compressibility.

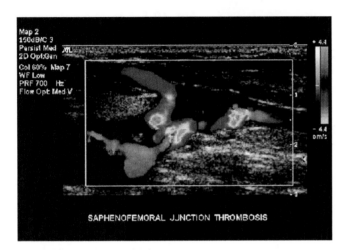

Fig. 10.7 *Color Doppler showing flow around an incompletely occlusive thrombus at the saphenofemoral junction.*

Diameter of the vein

- The diameter increases from the bulk of thrombus in the acute phase (Fig. 10.8).
- It then gradually shrinks to become smaller than normal in the chronic phase.

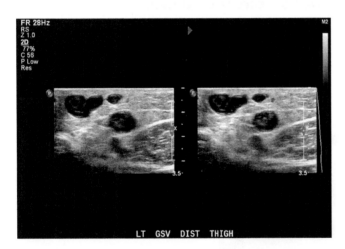

Fig. 10.8 *Superficial thrombophlebitis showing marked venous distension.*

Thickening of the vein wall

- The wall thickness gradually increases with time.

Criteria for diagnosing thrombosis – indirect evidence
Loss of phasic flow

- Loss of phasic flow with respiration or little or no response to the Valsalva maneuver (see chapter 11, page 206) in the CFV suggests obstruction proximal to the examination site.

- However, normal spectral Doppler cannot exclude DVT because there may be only partial thrombosis in the abdominal veins.
- Of the criteria, this requires the most experience.

Loss of change of diameter with the Valsalva maneuver

- No change in the CFV diameter suggests proximal occlusive thrombosis.

Minimal flow augmentation after calf compression

- This suggests occlusion between the examination and the augmentation sites.

Increased diameter and flow in superficial veins

- They enlarge if they are acting as collaterals.

Deep collaterals

- Large deep veins may be seen adjacent to the thrombosed vein, acting as collaterals.

NOTE!

- Deep veins always accompany their corresponding arteries and this helps to correctly identify deep veins rather than collaterals, particularly if chronic thrombosis has caused a vein to atrophy.

Ultrasound findings relating to the age of thrombus
Acute thrombus

- Loss of compressibility.
- Thrombus with low echogenicity.
- Increased vein diameter.
- Free-floating thrombus (Fig. 10.9).
- No flow on distal augmentation or the Valsalva maneuver.

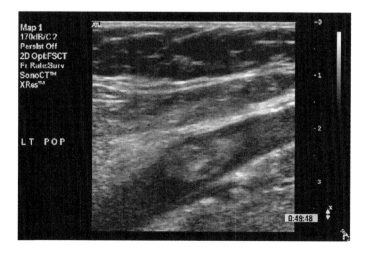

Fig. 10.9 *'Free-floating' thrombus in the popliteal vein.*

Subacute thrombus
- Lost or partial compressibility.
- Increased thrombus echogenicity.
- Reduced vein diameter.
- Thrombus adherent to wall.
- Recanalization.

Chronic thrombus
- Partial compressibility.
- Moderate-to-marked thrombus echogenicity.
- Reduced vein diameter – it may be atrophied.
- Collateral flow in the region.
- Recanalization.
- Thick vein wall.

PROTOCOLS FOR SCANNING

- Preparing the patient, selecting the best transducer, and general principles for scanning are discussed in Chapter 3 (pages 37–39).
- For all veins, the patient can lie flat or in reverse Trendelenberg* to ≥30° to help fill the veins for optimal scanning.
- Alter patient positioning to access veins with the least discomfort if the pain from venous thrombosis is intense.

WARNING!

- With repeated tests for surveillance after a DVT, ensure that levels for the extent of thrombus for each test are taken from the same bone, surface or confluence landmarks.

Groin veins
Position the patient and select windows
- Lay the patient supine with the affected leg externally rotated.
- Examine veins in the groin through the femoral triangle.

Scan the CFV, SFJ and femoral confluence
- Identify the CFV medial to the corresponding artery and also identify the SFJ.
- Use spectral Doppler in longitudinal to help distinguish the CFV from the artery.
- In transverse and B-mode, center the CFV in the image and compress with the transducer to assess if the CFV is fully compressible.
- Use B-mode and color Doppler to see if the vein is fully or partially thrombosed and whether thrombus is 'free floating.' Confirm with spectral Doppler.

---

*Friedrich Trendelenburg, 1844-1924, German surgeon

- In longitudinal, assess the CFV with color and spectral Doppler. Examine for phasicity with normal respiration and cessation of flow with the Valsalva maneuver to show that proximal veins are patent.
- Scan distally to identify the SFJ and the femoral confluence of the SFV and PFV. Test for compressibility and normal Doppler characteristics.
- In B-mode, measure thrombus extent and location from an anatomical landmark.
- Enlarged lymph nodes in the groin can be confused with a mass of thrombus but they can be distinguished because lymph nodes have closed ends.

NOTE!

- **Do not compress the vein any more than necessary if there has been recent thrombosis for fear of detaching thrombus to cause a PE.**

Thigh veins

Position the patient and select windows

- Continue with the patient lying in supine with the appropriate leg externally rotated.
- Examine deep veins in the thigh from an anteromedial approach.
- The GSV can easily be scanned through a medial window.
- Image quality may deteriorate as the FV passes through the adductor hiatus. Straighten the leg and use an anterior approach through vastus medialis; the vein is further from the transducer but the image is improved.

Scan the FV

- Use B-mode to identify the origin of the FV in transverse just as for the CFV and again test for compressibility.
- Continue down the FV to the distal thigh, in B-mode compress every 1–2 cm to test for compressibility.
- Use color Doppler at 1- to 2-cm intervals to show vein patency by augmentation after calf or distal thigh compression.
- If it is not certain that thrombus is present with B-mode and color Doppler, use spectral Doppler to confirm that there is no flow.
- When you reach the adductor hiatus, start working posteriorly and then return to a more anterior approach in the distal thigh.
- In B-mode, measure thrombus extent and location from the knee crease or inguinal ligament.

TIP!

- **It can be difficult to compress the distal FV when imaging through the anteromedial window. If so, place your free hand behind the thigh and push the limb into the transducer rather than trying to compress the vein through the anterior muscles.**

> **NOTE!**
>
> - Remember that the FV and the popliteal vein may be duplicated and both veins need to be assessed.
> - Adjacent arteries and nerves can be confused with veins during ultrasound examinations.

Scan the GSV above knee

- Use B-mode in transverse to check for compressibility of the GSV. Then use color Doppler to check for full color filling with distal augmentation.
- If the vein is incompressible, follow thrombus through the length of the GSV and major tributaries to the knee crease.
- If thrombus is identified, measure its extent and location from an anatomical landmark.

> **WARNING!**
>
> - Initially, do not press too hard because the normal vein collapses very easily, making it difficult to find.

Posterior veins

Position the patient and select windows

- Turn the patient prone or in lateral decubitus with the knee slightly flexed.
- Posterior windows are suitable.

Scan the popliteal vein, medial and lateral gastrocnemius veins, soleal sinuses and SSV

- Scan from behind the knee in B-mode and transverse to identify the single or paired popliteal vein which is usually superficial to the popliteal artery.
- As described above, assess the popliteal vein for compressibility and patency as far proximal as possible.
- As you reach the mid-popliteal vein, you will see several communications including the SSV and gastrocnemius veins. Extra force may be needed to compress the distal popliteal vein.
- As described above, examine the paired medial and lateral gastrocnemius veins from their confluence with the popliteal vein to as far down into the gastrocnemius muscles as possible.
- As described above, examine the soleal sinuses which are situated lower and deeper in the calf than the gastrocnemius veins. They are frequently visible only if distended with thrombus.
- View the SSV in this region and test for compressibility and patency down the posterior calf.
- If thrombus is identified, measure its extent and location from an anatomical landmark.
- Within the popliteal fossa, check for the presence and integrity of a Baker cyst (Fig. 10.10).

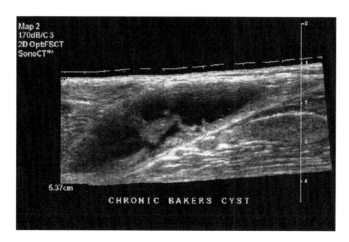

Fig. 10.10 A Baker's cyst in the popliteal fossa.

TIP!

- The gastrocnemius veins and soleal sinuses are common sites for thrombosis. They are always paired and often contain stagnant blood which may resemble fresh thrombus.

Calf veins
Position the patient and select windows

- The best method to view calf veins is to sit the patient on the side of the bed facing the sonographer with the foot on your knee to allow the calf muscles to drop away and better fill the veins.
- Scan from the medial or posteromedial aspect for the PTV and peroneal veins.
- The peroneal veins can also be seen through a posterior or anterolateral window.
- The below-knee GSV can be seen through a medial window.

Scan the tibial veins and distal GSV

- As described above, assess the GSV and tributaries below the knee and throughout the tibial veins for compressibility in B-mode and flow augmentation with color and spectral Doppler.
- Carefully examine for the presence of partial thrombus in the tibial veins.
- If thrombus is identified, measure the extent and location from the medial malleolus or knee crease.
- We consider that ATV thrombosis is so rare that it is not worth scanning these veins.

Abdominal veins
Position the patient and select windows

- Scan with the patient lying in supine.
- Image the IVC from an anterior approach through the rectus abdominis muscles to the right of the midline, superior to the umbilicus and at the umbilical level.

- The IVC can be viewed with the patient in left lateral decubitus and a coronal (flank) window if the patient is gassy or obese.
- Image from an oblique approach to separate the iliac veins and arteries.
- When technically difficult, the iliac veins can also be imaged with the patient in appropriate lateral decubitus positions.

Scan the IVC and iliac veins

- The examination should extend to assess these veins in patients with thrombus extending to the inguinal ligament or if flow patterns in the CFV suggest proximal occlusion.
- If iliac veins need to be examined, it is best to do this last because you will need to change to the lower frequency curved- or phased-array transducer for deeper penetration.
- It is difficult to compress abdominal veins.
- Use color Doppler to follow iliac veins to the IVC. Loss of color flow may suggest occlusive thrombus.
- Use spectral Doppler to confirm color findings of loss of flow. If flow is seen throughout the iliac veins and IVC, the veins are patent although they could still be partially thrombosed.
- If thrombus is present, note its extent.

ULTRASOUND IMAGES TO RECORD

- Transverse B-mode dual images to demonstrate compressibility of all superficial and deep veins
- Spectral trace in longitudinal for flow in the CFV with normal respiration and the Valsalva maneuver
- Spectral trace of all proximal veins during the Valsalva maneuver
- Spectral trace of all mid- to distal veins during distal augmentation
- Spectral traces and color Doppler images to demonstrate lack of flow in thrombosed veins.
- B-mode images of thrombus to determine age; note if thrombus is partially or fully occlusive.
- Note proximal and distal extents of all thrombi in relation to relevant anatomical landmarks
- Demonstrate other pathology such as lymphedema or a Baker's cyst.

WORKSHEET
Venous thrombosis in the lower limbs

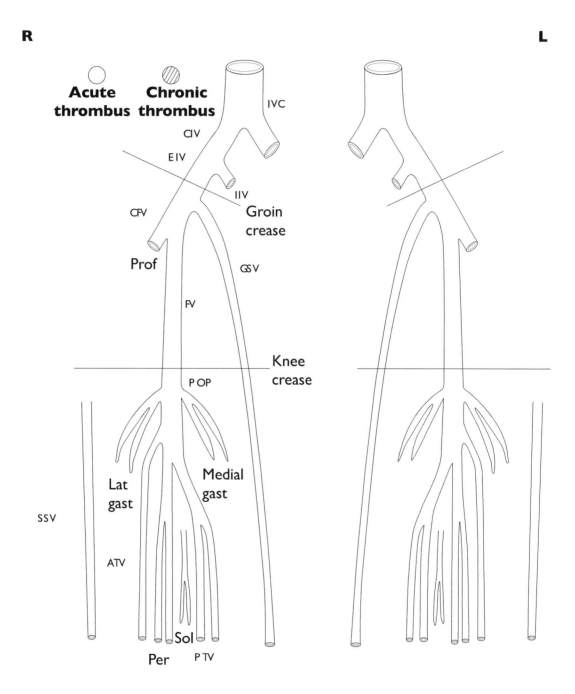

- Draw representation of thrombus and location.

CHRONIC VENOUS DISEASE IN THE LOWER LIMBS

Ultrasound for chronic venous disease detects connections between deep and superficial veins, reflux in deep and superficial veins, flow in perforator veins or venous obstruction. Continuous-wave Doppler supplements clinical assessment but duplex scanning is required to define anatomy. Computed tomography (CT) or magnetic resonance venography (MRV) may be required to show whether or not there is flow in the iliac veins and inferior vena cava (IVC).

ANATOMY

Veins scanned for reporting – all patients:
- Great saphenous vein (previously greater, long, internal) – GSV
- Small saphenous vein (previously lesser, short, external) – SSV
- Anterior and posterior accessory saphenous veins – AASV and PASV
- Anterior and posterior thigh circumflex veins (previously anterior and posterior thigh veins) – ATCV and PTCV
- Thigh extension of SSV – TE
- Vein of Giacomini*
- Saphenofemoral junction – SFJ
- Saphenopopliteal junction – SPJ
- Medial gastrocnemius veins
- Thigh and calf perforators
- Superficial tributaries
- Common femoral vein – CFV
- Profunda femoris vein – PFV
- Femoral vein (previously superficial femoral vein) – FV
- Popliteal vein
- Posterior tibial veins – PTV
- Peroneal veins.

Veins scanned for reporting – selected patients:
- Inferior vena cava (IVC)
- Common, internal and external iliac veins – CIV, IIV, EIV
- Ovarian veins
- Anterior tibial veins – ATV
- Lateral gastrocnemius and soleal veins.

- A service may use different terminology, which must be made clear if abbreviations are used.
- The anatomy of deep veins is discussed in Chapter 10.
- The terminology is that recommended by the International Union of Phlebology (Cavezzi et al. 2006**).

---

*Carlo Giacomini, 1840–1898, Professor of Anatomy at University of Turin, Italy

** Cavezzi A, Labropoulos N, Partsch H, et al. Duplex ultrasound investigation of the veins in chronic venous disease of the lower limbs – UIP consensus document. Part II. Anatomy. *Eur J Vasc Endovasc Surg* 2006;**31**:288

GSV and AASV (Fig. 11.1)
Relation of GSV to superficial fascia (Fig. 11.2)
- The SFJ position is constant just lateral to the pubic tubercle.
- The GSV lies within a superficial compartment formed by the deep and superficial fascias – the 'saphenous eye'.
- All tributaries including the ATCV and PTCV lie superficial to the superficial fascia.

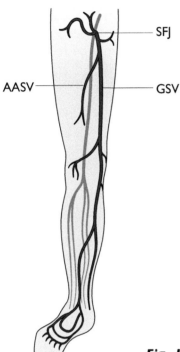

Fig. 11.1 *Anatomy of the GSV and AASV in the right lower limb.*

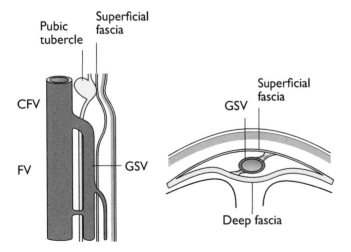

a

Fig. 11.2 *GSV – relation to superficial fascia:*
a *Redrawn from Fig. 1, Caggiati A. Phlebology 1997;**12**:107, with permission from the Royal Society of Medicine Press, London.*

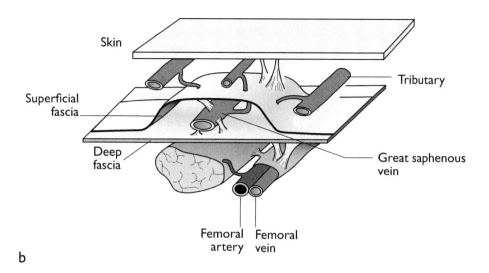

b

Fig. 11.2 (continued)

b *Reprinted from Fig. 1, Caggiati A, Bergan A, Gloviczki P et al. J Vasc Surg 2002;**36**:416 with permission from the Society for Vascular Surgery.*

Variations of GSV in the thigh (Fig. 11.3)

- GSV present to the knee:
  - No major tributaries (Fig. 11.3a).
  - GSV duplicated – one compartment – very uncommon (Fig. 11.3b).
  - Major tributary that joins above the knee (Fig. 11.3c).
  - GSV duplicated – two compartments (Fig. 11.3d).
- GSV not present at the knee:
  - Absence of variable length of GSV above knee (Fig. 11.3e).

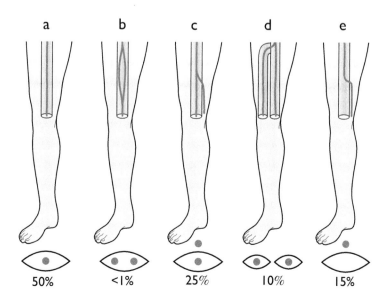

Fig. 11.3 *GSV – variations in the thigh.*

*Redrawn from Fig. 1, Ricci S. Phlebology 2002;**16**:111 with permission from the Royal Society of Medicine Press, London.*

Variations of GSV in the distal thigh and calf (Fig. 11.4)

- GSV present at the knee (70%):
  - No major tributaries (Fig. 11.4a).
  - Major tributaries below the knee (Fig. 11.4b).
  - Major tributary above the knee (Fig. 11.4c).
- GSV not present at the knee (30%):
  - Absence of considerable length of GSV above the knee (Fig. 11.4d).
  - Absence of short length of GSV at and below the knee (Fig. 11.4e).

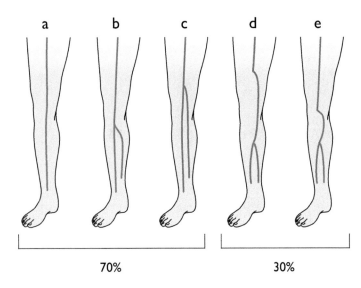

Fig. 11.4 *GSV – variations in the distal thigh and calf.*

*Redrawn from Fig. 2, Ricci S. Phlebology 1999;**14**:59 with permission from the Royal Society of Medicine Press, London.*

Variations in the origin of the AASV (Fig. 11.5)

- Common junction with GSV (Fig. 11.5a).
- Origin from GSV below the SFJ (Fig. 11.5b).
- Origin from CFV above the SFJ (Fig. 11.5c).
- Origin from the SFJ as principal vein with hypoplastic or absent GSV (Fig. 11.5d).

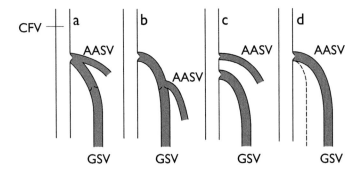

Fig. 11.5 *AASV – variations in its origin.*

SSV and TE (Fig. 11.6)

- The SSV may be in the midline or medial or lateral to the midline.
- The TE is present in 95% of limbs and is the continuation of the SSV.

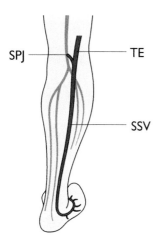

Fig. 11.6 *Anatomy of the small saphenous vein in the right lower limb.*

Variations in its termination (Fig. 11.7)

- The SSV may join the popliteal vein or deep veins at a higher level (Fig. 11.7a).
- There may be no connection to deep veins (Fig. 11.7b).

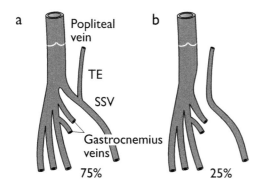

Fig. 11.7 *SSV – variations in its termination.*

Level of the SPJ (Fig. 11.8)

- The level is variable.
- It is most often 2–4 cm above the knee crease.
- Twenty-five percent are higher than this level.
- The junction is rarely below the knee crease.

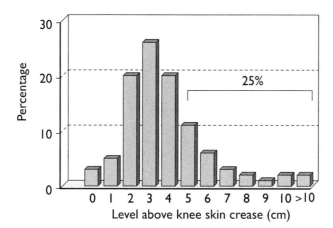

Fig. 11.8 *SSV – level of SPJ from our studies.*

Perforators (Fig. 11.9)

- They pass through the deep fascia to connect deep and superficial veins.
- A valve normally directs flow from superficial to deep.
- Thigh perforators usually pass from the GSV to the FV.
- Calf perforators can pass from the GSV, SSV or major tributaries to tibial veins, or to calf muscle venous plexus.
- In order of frequency, calf perforators are on the medial, posterior, lateral or anterior aspects.

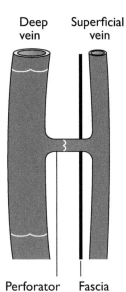

Deep vein   Superficial vein

Perforator   Fascia

Fig. 11.9 *Perforators.*

CLINICAL ASPECTS

Regional pathology

- Varicose veins: large veins that bulge above the skin surface usually affecting saphenous vein tributaries.
- Reticular veins: smaller blue veins that do not protrude.
- Telangiectases: tiny short unconnected or spidery branching vessels.

Primary superficial venous disease

- From our studies, we found the following patterns of reflux through connections to the GSV in males and females:

	Females (%)	Males (%)
SFJ	55	80
Low pelvic/abdominal veins	35	10
Perforators	3	3
Unknown	7	7

- From our studies, we found the following patterns of reflux through connections to the SSV:

SPJ	65%
GSV tributaries	15%
TE	15%
Popliteal perforators	5%

- From our studies, we found the following proximal terminations for the TE and vein of Giacomini:
  - ○ PTCV to GSV (vein of Giacomini)   70%
  - ○ Abdominal or pelvic veins   15%
  - ○ FV   10%
  - ○ Deep veins in buttock   5%

- In addition, flow in the TE and vein of Giacomini could be in either direction:
  - ○ Downward flow from the GSV, pelvic veins or deep veins through the TE to the SSV.
  - ○ Upward flow from the SSV through the TE or vein of Giacomini to the GSV.

Recurrent superficial venous disease after treatment

- Appreciable numbers of patients develop recurrent varicose veins after any form of treatment due to the following causes:
  - ○ Residual veins in the treated territory that were not eliminated at the time.
  - ○ True recurrence in the venous territory of veins that were previously treated.
  - ○ New varicose veins in a territory other than that previously treated.
- Patterns of reflux for recurrent varicose veins are even more complex than for untreated disease.
- Recurrence after treatment for GSV reflux affects the GSV territory in two-thirds or results from new disease with SSV or perforator reflux in one-third.
- Frequently, there are multiple deep to superficial connections.
- Similar considerations apply to the SPJ after SSV treatment where veins from the popliteal fossa connect to the SSV or calf tributaries.
- From our studies, we found the following patterns of reflux through connections to the GSV for recurrent varicose veins:
  - ○ SFJ   25%
  - ○ Low pelvic/abdominal veins   50%
  - ○ Perforators   15%
  - ○ Unknown   10%

Deep venous disease

- Deep venous disease may involve occlusion, reflux or both.
- Deep venous occlusion may be acquired from past thrombosis with incomplete or failed recanalization (Fig. 11.10) or it may be congenital or primary.

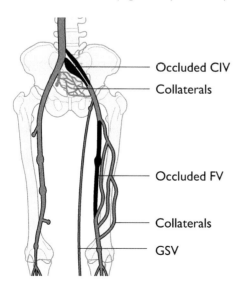

Occluded CIV

Collaterals

Occluded FV

Collaterals

GSV

Fig. 11.10 *Long-standing occlusion of the FV or EIV and CIV.*
- *There is flow through superficial veins acting as collaterals.*

From Fig. 11.8, Myers KA, Marshall RD, Freidin J. Principles of Pathology. Oxford: Blackwell, 1980. Reproduced with permission from Blackwell.

- The degree to which flow is restricted depends on the extent of occlusion, where it is situated, the presence of a duplicated vein and the amount of collateral flow.
- Deep venous reflux may involve the full length of the limb or isolated venous segments.
- We define deep reflux as being present if it extends beyond the valve below either junction.
- Brief reverse flow over a short deep segment with no superficial reflux is assumed to be normal flow between valves.
- A short segment of reflux in the CFV opposite an incompetent SFJ, and in the popliteal vein opposite an incompetent SPJ is not a pathological deep reflux but simply blood passing to the superficial veins.
- The amplitude and duration of deep reflux do not relate to the severity of varicose veins or risk of complications.

Clinical presentations
Complications of chronic venous disease
- Complications are frequently referred to as the 'post-thrombotic syndrome' implying that they are inevitably a consequence of past deep vein thrombosis (DVT) and recanalization or obstruction.
- However, duplex scanning has shown that many patients develop complications from superficial reflux alone.
- Venous hypertension can damage skin and fat causing lipodermatosclerosis which can lead to venous eczema or ulceration (Fig. 11.11), particularly at the ankle.
- Deep venous obstruction can cause 'venous claudication' which is bursting pain in the calf during exercise relieved by leg elevation.

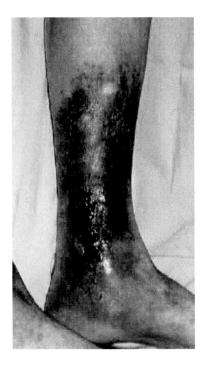

Fig. 11.11 *Lipodermatosclerosis, pigmentation, venous eczema and ulceration at the medial ankle.*

CEAP classification

This is used to characterize venous disease:

- *C – Clinical* classification:
  - C 0   No visible or palpable signs of venous disease.
  - C 1   Telangiectases or reticular veins.
  - C 2   Varicose veins.
  - C 3   Edema.
  - C 4   Skin changes ascribed to venous disease:
    - A – pigmentation or eczema.
    - B – lipodermatosclerosis or atrophy blanche.
  - C 5   Skin changes with healed ulcer.
  - C 6   Skin changes with active ulcer.
- *E – Etiologic* classification:
  - Ec   Congenital problems apparent at birth or recognized later.
  - Ep   Primary problems that are not congenital with no identifiable cause.
  - Es   Secondary problems that are acquired with known pathology such as post-thrombotic or post-traumatic.
- *A – Anatomic* classification.
  - As   Superficial veins:
    - 1   Telangiectases and reticular veins
    - 2   GSV above the knee
    - 3   GSV below the knee
    - 4   SSV
    - 5   Non-saphenous
  - Ad   Deep veins:
    - 6   IVC
    - 7   CIV
    - 8   IIV
    - 9   EIV
    - 10   Pelvic – gonadal, broad ligament
    - 11   CFV
    - 12   PFV
    - 13   FV
    - 14   Popliteal
    - 15   Crural – ATV, PTV, peroneal
    - 16   Muscular – gastrocnemial, soleal, other
  - Ap   Perforator veins:
    - 17   Thigh
    - 18   Calf
- *P – Pathophysiological* classification:
  - Pr   Reflux
  - Po   Obstruction
  - Pro   Both

- Patients present for cosmetic reasons or with symptoms that are not necessarily proportional to the size of their veins.
- Many symptoms are due to conditions other than varicose veins.
- Athletes' prominent veins are not a clinical problem.
- Large dilated veins can appear in pregnancy and often regress after delivery.

Differential diagnosis
- Aching pain with walking or ulceration due to occlusive arterial disease.
- Swelling from lymphedema.
- Skin changes from cellulitis.

Treatment
- Conservative treatment with compression may be preferred.
- Diameters have become important to help select best treatment.
- Injection sclerotherapy is used for smaller visible veins.
- Ultrasound-guided sclerotherapy is preferred for small- to medium-sized saphenous veins or tributaries (see Chapter 15).
- Surgery or endovenous ablation may be preferred for reflux in larger-diameter veins (see Chapter 15).
- Surgery for either saphenous vein combines variations of three techniques:
  - Ligation at the saphenous junction including all tributaries in the region.
  - Stripping a length of the saphenous vein. Due to proximity to surface sensory nerves, many limit stripping to the GSV between the groin and knee and the SSV to just behind the knee.
  - Avulsion phlebectomy of superficial tributaries through multiple tiny punctures.

> **NOTE!**
> - Surface varicose veins affecting tributaries can be seen and it is not necessary to describe them in detail by duplex scanning.

CLINICAL ASPECTS – OTHER VENOUS DISEASES

Hemangiomas, venous malformations and Klippel–Trenaunay syndrome
- See Chapter 12.

Left common iliac vein compression (May–Thurner syndrome) (Fig. 11.12)
- This occurs if the right common iliac artery compresses the left CIV as the artery becomes more rigid and tortuous with age (described by R May and J Thurner in 1957*).

Popliteal vein entrapment
- The vein is trapped by the gastrocnemius when the knee is extended and can cause calf pain or predispose to DVT.
- However, it is also commonly observed in individuals with no venous disease.

Venous aneurysms
- These are uncommon but can affect the popliteal or femoral vein.
- They are saccular or fusiform and usually lined by thrombus.
- They have a high risk of pulmonary embolism.

---

* R. May, J. Thurner, The cause of the predominantly sinistral occurrence of thrombosis of the pelvic veins. *Angiology*, 1957, 8: 419–427

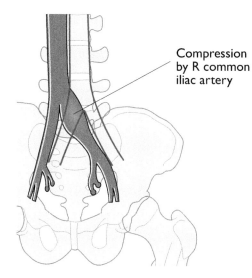

Compression
by R common
iliac artery

Fig. 11.12 *May–Thurner syndrome – compression of the left common iliac vein by the right common iliac artery.*

From Fig. 11.7a, Myers KA, Marshall RD, Freidin J. Principles of Pathology. Oxford: Blackwell, 1980. Reproduced with permission from Blackwell.

WHAT DOCTORS NEED TO KNOW

- Are there sites of refluxing connections from deep to superficial veins through the saphenous junctions, incompetent perforators or other veins?
- Is there superficial venous reflux in the GSV or SSV and their tributaries?
- What is the extent of GSV or SSV affected by reflux?
- What are the diameters of incompetent saphenous junctions, saphenous veins and perforators?
- Is the SPJ present and what is its level?
- Is there reflux in veins such as the TE, vein of Giacomini or gastrocnemius veins?
- Is there deep venous reflux or obstruction?

THE DUPLEX SCAN

Indications for scanning
- Primary uncomplicated varicose veins in GSV territory.
- Primary uncomplicated varicose veins in SSV territory.
- Recurrent varicose veins.
- Chronic venous disease with skin complications.
- Symptoms of venous disease without evidence of varicose veins.
- Surveillance after treatment.
- Marking the site before surgery for varicose veins.
- Marking the location and diameter before using GSV for femoropopliteal or coronary artery bypass grafting.

Normal findings
- Reflux is flow in veins away from the heart and is normally prevented by valves.
- There is transient reflux for ≤0.5 s as normal valves close.

Criteria for venous reflux
- The original definition of reflux was reverse flow for >0.5 s, but many consider that reflux for >1 s is required.

- Ultrasound should demonstrate deep to superficial connections for reflux into superficial veins but this is not possible in approximately 10%.

PROTOCOLS FOR SCANNING

- Preparing the patient, selecting the best transducer, and general principles for scanning are discussed in Chapter 3 (pages 37–39).
- For all veins, scan with the patient standing or tilted on a table in reverse Trendelenburg to >45°.

NOTE!

- Reflux is more likely to develop later in the day and in a warm environment.
- A cold environment can cause veins to constrict and make them difficult to see and in some cases causes refluxing veins to apparently become competent.
- These may change results of scans in patients with borderline reflux.

Eliciting reflux

- We prefer to elicit reflux in proximal veins by the Valsalva* maneuver (Fig. 11.13). This results from forced expiration against a closed glottis. The patient is asked to take a deep breath and then strain for a few seconds while holding the breath.
- Others prefer compression and then release with a thigh or calf squeeze for proximal veins or calf or foot squeeze for calf veins (Fig. 11.14).
- Use manual compression of varicose vein clusters.
- Use pneumatic calf cuff deflation.
- Use active foot dorsiflexion and relaxation.

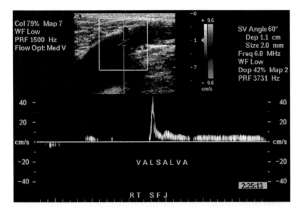

Fig. 11.13 Spectral Doppler for reflux at the SFJ produced by the Valsalva maneuver.

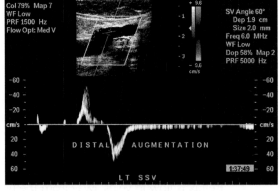

Fig. 11.14 Spectral Doppler for reflux at the SPJ produced by augmentation.
- Anterograde flow in the SSV with calf compression followed by retrograde flow after release of calf compression.

*Antonio Maria Valsalva, 1666–1723, Italian anatomist

Other considerations
- Scan both limbs at the first examination.
- The skin position in relation to veins changes with movement from upright to supine.
- If veins are being marked with an indelible pen before surgery or endovenous ablation, this should be performed with the patient supine and the limb in the operation position.

TIPS!
- The best way to assess varicose veins is to initially ignore varicosities and scan for sites of incompetence feeding to these veins. Only if this fails to show connections should varices be traced back to the saphenous veins.
- To minimize scan time, look for perforators while testing for deep and superficial reflux.
- Transducer pressure should remain light to ensure that superficial veins are not compressed making it difficult for them to be seen or causing incompetent veins to become apparently competent.
- Do not be afraid to rest your scanning arm on the patient so that transducer pressure can be kept light without causing the sonographer muscle strain.

Veins above the knee
Position the patient and select windows
- If standing, the patient faces towards the sonographer with the leg being examined rotated outwards and the weight taken on the opposite leg.
- If on a tilt bed, lay the patient supine with the affected leg externally rotated.
- Examine the veins in the groin through the femoral triangle.
- The GSV can easily be scanned through a medial window.
- The AASV can be seen through an anterior window.
- Examine the deep veins in the thigh from an anteromedial approach.
- Image quality may deteriorate as the FV passes through the adductor hiatus. Straighten the leg and use an anterior approach through vastus medialis. The vein is further from the transducer but the image is improved.

Scan the GSV and AASV above the knee
- Commence in the groin in transverse to show the SFJ and CFV as the 'Mickey Mouse sign' (see Fig. 3.7A). If the junction is not present due to ligation of the GSV, then 'Mickey's' medial ear is missing.
- If present, determine connections for reflux by spectral or color Doppler from SFJ incompetence, veins from the low abdomen or pelvis, thigh or calf perforators or the vein of Giacomini.
- In transverse, determine whether the destination for reflux is into the GSV or the major thigh tributaries. Measure the level of inflow of reflux to the GSV if it is distal to the SFJ.
- Scan for saphenous reflux distal to communication with a significant tributary (diameter >4 mm).
- Suspect a connection for reflux if there is a sudden increase in GSV diameter, although diameters decrease below major refluxing tributaries.

- Follow the full length of GSV and tributaries to the knee. Test every few centimeters for compressibility and reflux.
- Measure diameters at the junction and along the GSV and AASV if there is reflux.

TIP!

- *'The alignment sign'*: The GSV and AASV can be distinguished by ultrasound from their relation to the femoral artery and vein (Fig. 11.15).

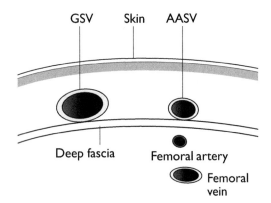

Fig. 11.15 *Alignment sign in the left lower limb.*
- *The AASV lies superficial to the femoral artery and vein. The GSV is more medial.*

Scan the CFV, PFV and FV

- Test the CFV in longitudinal with spectral Doppler for phasicity with normal respiration, cessation of flow with deep inspiration, and reflux with the Valsalva maneuver. Lack of phasicity may indicate proximal obstruction and the ultrasound should be extended later to show the iliac veins and the IVC.
- Test the femoral confluence for reflux or thrombosis.
- Follow the full length of FV to the above-knee popliteal vein testing for reflux or thrombosis.
- Slow outflow during distal compression suggests occlusion between the test and augmentation sites.
- Record spectral traces.

Scan the thigh perforators

- Perforators pass through the deep fascia which is a distinct hyperechoic band on B-mode (Fig. 11.16).
- Use color Doppler to test for outward flow in perforators by thigh muscle contraction. Use spectral Doppler if flow direction and duration are ambiguous.
- Scan for perforators on the medial thigh as the full length of the GSV and deep veins are examined.
- Look for lateral, posterior and anterior thigh perforators if clinical assessment shows varices in these regions.
- Measure the levels of refluxing perforators from the inguinal ligament or skin crease behind the knee and measure their diameters with B-mode.
- Record spectral traces.

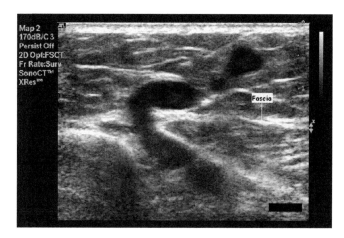

Fig. 11.16 *A perforator passing through the deep fascia shown by B-mode.*

NOTE!

● Insonate the fascia at 90° to ensure maximum specular reflection to help identify perforators passing through the fascia.

Posterior veins of thigh and calf
Position the patient and select windows
● Turn the patient prone or in lateral decubitus with the knee slightly flexed.
● Turn the patient to face away from the sonographer if standing.
● Posterior windows are suitable.

Scan the SSV, TE and vein of Giacomini
● Start at the back of the knee.
● Determine whether the SPJ is present. If so, insonate the junction in longitudinal.
● Determine if there is SPJ incompetence with SSV reflux.
● Look for alternate connections for reflux including communication with popliteal fossa perforators, GSV tributaries, pelvic veins traced to the buttock or perineum, TE or vein of Giacomini.
● Look for alternate connections for SSV reflux, including tributaries, TE or vein of Giacomini.
● Examine the TE and vein of Giacomini. Determine the distal SSV connection and proximal connection into the GSV or the deep or pelvic veins.
● If there is reflux, measure diameters at the SPJ and along the SSV, TE and vein of Giacomini.
● Record spectral traces.
● Measure the level of the SPJ in relation to the skin crease behind the knee.

Scan the popliteal vein and medial gastrocnemius veins
● Test the popliteal vein for reflux or thrombosis proximal and distal to the SPJ.
● Test the medial gastrocnemius veins for reflux or thrombosis.
● Record spectral traces.

Veins below the knee
Position the patient and select windows
- The best method to view infrapopliteal veins is to sit the patient on the side of the bed facing the sonographer with the foot on the sonographer's knee to allow the calf muscles to drop away and better fill veins.
- The GSV can be imaged from a medial approach.
- Scan from the medial or posteromedial aspect for the PTV and peroneal veins.
- The peroneal veins can also be seen through a posterior or anterolateral window.

GSV below the knee
- Determine whether the below-knee GSV is present.
- Continue down its length as for the above-knee GSV.
- Examine for reflux and thrombosis.
- Measure diameters in B-mode if reflux present.
- Record spectral traces.

TIP!
- 'The tibio–gastrocnemius angle sign' is useful to detect the GSV at the knee (Fig. 11.17).

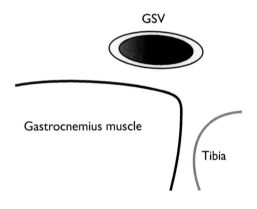

Fig. 11.17 Tibio–gastrocnemius angle sign.
- If the GSV is present at the knee, it lies superficial to the angle of gastrocnemius just behind the tibia.

Tibial veins
- Examine for reflux or thrombosis throughout the PTVs and peroneal veins.
- Record spectral traces.

NOTE!
- With experience, all tibial veins can be identified.
- Reflux in the PTV best reflects clinical features.
- It is optional to scan the ATV.

Calf perforators

- Test for outward flow by color Doppler after a calf muscle squeeze, isometric calf muscle contraction or foot squeeze. Wait for >15 s to allow calf muscles to refill before repeating the squeeze. Use spectral Doppler if flow direction and duration are ambiguous with color Doppler (Fig. 11.18).
- Look for perforators around the calf circumference. If they show outward flow, measure their level from the medial or lateral malleolus and use B-mode to measure their diameters at the deep fascia.
- Record spectral traces.

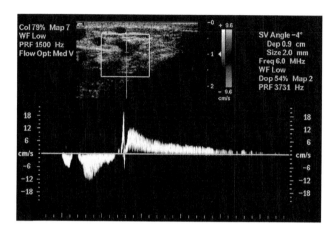

Fig. 11.18 *Outward flow in a calf perforator shown by spectral Doppler.*

Abdominal veins

Position the patient and select windows

- With the patient supine, image the IVC from an anterior approach through rectus abdominis to the right of the midline, superior to the umbilicus and at the umbilical level.
- The IVC can be viewed from the right lateral decubitus position if the patient is gassy or obese.
- The ovarian veins are best seen with the patient in supine with an anterior window.
- Image from an oblique approach to separate the iliac veins and arteries.
- When technically difficult, the iliac veins can also be imaged with the patient in appropriate lateral decubitus positions.

Scan the IVC, and iliac and ovarian veins

- Scanning these veins is usually left until last if performed at all.
- Ovarian vein reflux, usually on the left, may be the connection through the pelvic veins into the legs in many women.
- Ovarian vein reflux is usually spontaneous.
- Iliac veins usually have no valves. Reflux may be detected into tributaries of the IIV or EIV.
- For the left side, find the left renal vein as it crosses the aorta and trace it out to where it is joined by the left ovarian vein passing vertically upwards.
- For the right side, find the IVC and trace it down to where the right ovarian vein joins it at an angle.
- Test for reflux either spontaneous or induced by epigastric compression. If spontaneous reflux is observed, this can be arrested by iliac fossa compression.
- If ovarian vein reflux is demonstrated, measure diameters in the proximal and distal segments.

- Use color Doppler to scan the pelvic floor looking for varicosities.
- Test the iliac veins for incompetence.
- Record spectral traces.

Scan for recurrent varicose veins

- These are the most difficult studies for varicose veins.
- Patterns of reflux are frequently different to primary varicose veins so be aware of the many possible sites.
- If there has been previous surgery to the GSV, examine the medial and posterior thigh for recurrence of a refluxing GSV and connections for reflux from CFV, pelvic, round ligament, gluteal, abdominal, ovarian, or pudendal tributaries or thigh perforators.
- After past surgery to the SSV, examine the popliteal fossa for connections at the SPJ, from popliteal or posterior calf perforators or from the TE or vein of Giacomini.
- Examine the leg for recurrence through calf perforators.

Scan for surveillance after treatment for varicose veins

- If the GSV and SSV are present, they should be examined throughout their lengths for thrombus, sclerosis or reflux.
- Scanning should include venous mapping and a complete DVT examination.
- Mark for location and diameters before use of GSV for femoropopliteal bypass graft or coronary artery bypass graft
- With an indelible pen, mark the course of the GSV on the skin.
- Note and mark levels of GSV diameter <3 mm on the skin.
- Note and mark areas of partial thrombus or wall thickening on the skin.
- Note and mark levels of large tributaries and perforators communicating with the GSV on the skin that may need to be ligated.

THE CONTINUOUS-WAVE DOPPLER EXAMINATION

- The hand-held continuous-wave (CW) Doppler can be used to assess each GSV and SSV system and the deep veins.
- Many doctors consider this to be a routine part of the clinical examination.

Examination for the GSV

- Stand the patient facing you with the knee slightly bent, heel on the ground, and weight on the opposite leg.
- Listen in the groin for the common femoral artery pulse. Move the probe a little medially to listen for reflux in the CFV after squeezing the calf.
- Move the probe a little more medial and down to be over the GSV, and listen for reflux after squeezing the calf. If there is reflux, then repeat and use a finger of the free hand to occlude the GSV below the probe to determine whether this stops reflux.
- Repeat, listening over a distal varicosity to determine whether there is reflux and whether this can be stopped by pressure over the GSV. To detect whether a varicosity and the GSV are connected, push on one while listening over the other with the CW transducer to hear . if there is a signal.

Examination for the SSV

- Stand the patient on a step facing away with the knee slightly bent, heel on the step and weight on the opposite leg.
- Sit behind the patient and listen for the popliteal artery signal. Move the probe to the SSV just lateral to the arterial signal, squeeze the calf and listen for reflux after releasing the squeeze.
- If there is reflux, repeat and use a finger of the free hand to occlude the SSV below the probe to determine whether this stops reflux.

ULTRASOUND IMAGES TO RECORD

- Sample spectral traces of proximal veins and SFJ in longitudinal with the Valsalva maneuver.
- Sample spectral traces of more distal veins and SPJ in longitudinal during augmentation and release.
- Sample spectral traces of reflux in other veins such as the AASV, TE, vein of Giacomini and gastrocnemius veins.
- B-mode for diameter of incompetent junctions; note the level of the SPJ from the knee crease.
- B-mode for maximum and minimum vein diameters in transverse if reflux is demonstrated in any saphenous vein.
- B-mode for diameters at the fascial border in transverse if there is outward flow in perforators; note locations from anatomical landmarks.
- Other pathology such as a Baker's cyst.

WORKSHEET
Chronic venous study

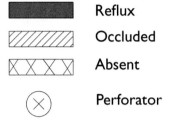

■ Reflux

▨ Occluded

▧ Absent

⊗ Perforator

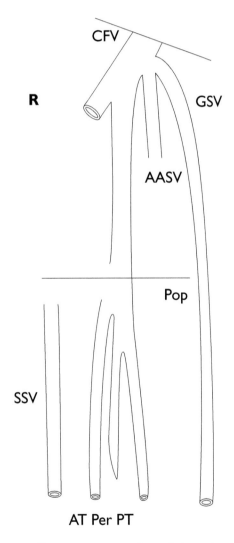

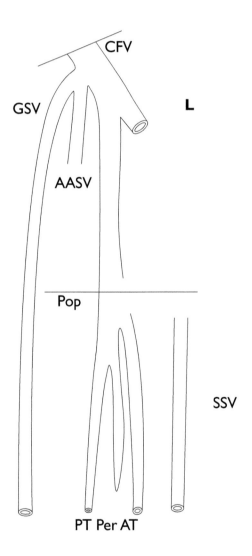

- Draw representation of thrombus and location.
- Draw representation of reflux in deep and saphenous veins.
- Draw representation of varicose veins.
- If present, draw SPj and note level.

12 VASCULAR TUMORS, MALFORMATIONS AND FISTULAS

Written and illustrated in association with Kurosh Parsi, Sydney, Australia

There is a wide variety of vascular tumors and congenital vascular malformations (CVMs). Their diagnosis and treatment can be difficult. Various imaging modalities are required for baseline evaluation and diagnosis including ultrasound examination, frequently followed by magnetic resonance imaging (MRI) or MR venography (MRV). Acquired arteriovenous fistulas (AVFs) result from trauma or disease and are well demonstrated by ultrasound. Surgically created AVFs for hemodialysis are discussed in Chapter 13.

CLINICAL ASPECTS – VASCULAR TUMORS

Hemangiomas
Etiology and pathology
- Hemangiomas are the most common vascular tumors.
- They can be congenital or appear during infancy (HOI – hemangioma of infancy).
- Subgroups of congenital hemangiomas:
    - Undergo rapid involution after birth; RICH is a rapidly involuting congenital hemangioma
    - Persist indefinitely; NICH is a non-involuting congenital hemangioma.
- What are commonly referred to as hemangiomas are actually HOIs.
- HOIs are the most common tumors of infancy and occur in approximately 10% of white people, more frequently in females.
- HOIs have three stages: initial proliferation and growth, a rest stage then involution.
- HOIs are 'self-limited' and benign.
- They consist of endothelial cells and are highly vascular.
- They are distinct from CVMs which are congenital and 'self-perpetuating'.

Clinical features
- Approximately 80% of HOIs are located on the face and neck (Fig. 12.1).
- The greatest concern is their appearance.
- Those on the surface have a 'strawberry' appearance whereas those under the skin present as a bluish swelling.
- Complications are uncommon but include surface ulceration and bleeding, pressure on vital organs or high-output cardiac failure if very large.

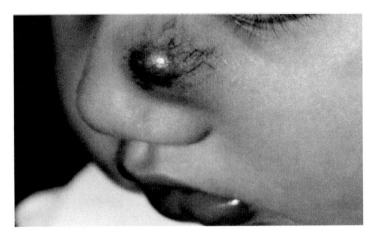

Fig. 12.1 *Clinical appearance of an HOI of the face.*

Treatment
- HOIs commonly disappear without treatment by 10 years of age leaving few or no visible marks.
- Large unsightly tumors or those causing complications require treatment.
- Topical or systemic β blocker drugs are most effective although surgical excision may be required.

Angiosarcomas
- These are rare malignant tumors with several variations.

CLINICAL ASPECTS – CVMs

Embryology
- The reticular phase occurs for the first 3 weeks of development.
- At this stage, the circulation consists of unstructured tangled small vessels actively growing from mesenchymal cells or angioblasts.
- Abnormalities of development that occur before the vascular system matures retain the active growing characteristics of these cells.
- After about 3 weeks, the vessels differentiate to form vascular trunks adjacent to the major nerves.
- Extratruncular or pretruncular lesions are due to arrested development in the reticular phase.
- Truncular lesions are due to later arrested development during the phase of vascular trunk formation.

Pathology
- Extratruncular malformations keep the characteristics of mesenchymal cells which allow them to grow if stimulated.
- They have an unpredictable course with a tendency to convert from a dormant to an active phase if provoked by trauma, hormones or especially surgical or non-surgical treatment.
- They have a high tendency to progress with destructive potential and a high recurrence rate and risk of complications.

- Truncular malformations can recur but lack the proliferative potential of extratruncular lesions.
- Truncular malformations are more hemodynamically significant than extratruncular malformations.

Classification for CVMs

- These are defined by the predominant malformation:
  - Venous malformation (VM).
  - Lymphatic malformation (LM).
  - Capillary malformation (CM).
  - Arteriovenous malformation (AVM).
  - Combined vascular malformations.
- The Hamburg Classification* avoids eponymous nomenclature but some syndrome names persist.

Embryological subclassification
Extratruncular forms
- Diffuse, infiltrating.
- Localized, limited.

Truncular forms
- Aplasia or obstruction:
  - Hypoplasia, aplasia, hyperplasia.
  - Stenosis, obstruction, congenital spur, membrane.
- Dilation:
  - Localized aneurysm.
  - Diffuse ectasia.

Presentations of CVM

- There is a wide range of presentations with unpredictable outcomes.
- Eight-five percent are asymptomatic.
- They may involve any organ system but most commonly they involve the pelvis, extremities and intracranial circulation.
- Most CVMs are VMs, LMs or CMs.
- AVMs are less common but are the most aggressive.

Venous malformations (Fig. 12.2)
Presentation and clinical features
- Extratruncular VMs present with multiple lesions in various tissues such as skin, fat and muscle.
- Extratruncular VMs can present as varicose veins, lesions or a lump or swelling depending on the tissue involved.
- Truncular VMs can closely mimic varicose veins.
- Extensive VMs can result in chronic venous insufficiency or superficial thrombophlebitis.
- Truncular VMs include the following:
  - Popliteal vein aneurysm.
  - Persistent sciatic or marginal vein.
  - Congenital deep vein incompetence.
  - Klippel–Trenaunay syndrome.

---

*The Hamburg Classification: based on a workshop held in Hamburg, Germany in 1988

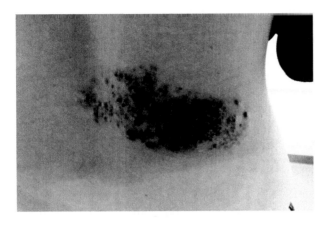

Fig. 12.2 *Clinical appearance of a VM of the back.*

- *Klippel–Trenaunay syndrome** (Fig. 12.3) is defined by the following features:
  - A combined capillary-lymphatic-venous malformation.
  - Not all three vascular components are always present.
  - Atypical, mostly lateral varicosities.
  - Soft-tissue and skeletal hypertrophy.
  - Involvement of one or more limbs and sometimes the trunk.
  - Overgrowth of one limb, usually the leg.

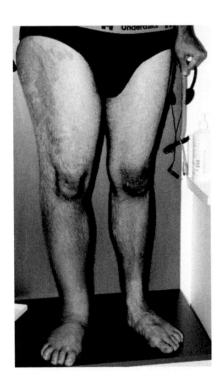

Fig. 12.3 *Clinical appearance of a leg in a patient with Klippel–Trenaunay syndrome.*

Modalities for diagnosis
- Initial assessment with continuous-wave Doppler to determine basic flow characteristics.
- Duplex ultrasound.

---

*Maurice Klippel and Paul Trenaunay, French physicians – described in 1900

- MRI to establish the extent.
- MRV to determine the feeding and draining vessels.
- Biopsy to determine the type of VM such as glomovenous malformation or blue rubber bleb syndrome.
- Genetic studies.

Treatment
- General measures such as graduated compression stockings.
- Endovenous laser ablation and foam ultrasound-guided sclerotherapy.
- Limited treatment options for deep vein incompetence.
- Surgery is rarely required for treatment of extratruncular lesions. Discrete lesions can be excised but frequently recur.

Lymphatic malformations (Fig. 12.4)
Presentation and clinical features
- Extratruncular LMs present with cystic lesions.
- Extratruncular LMs can present in two forms:
  - Microcystic: appear as a cluster of small warts or blisters.
  - Macrocystic: appear as lumps.
- The cysts can contain clear or blood-stained fluid. The vessel walls are fragile and minor trauma can result in bleeding into the cystic space.
- Truncular LMs present with primary lymphedema.
- LMs can present with recurrent cellulitis or other forms of localized infections.

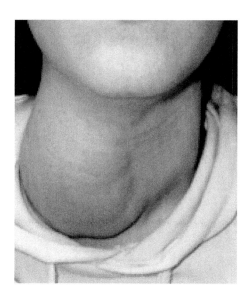

Fig. 12.4 *Clinical appearance of an LM of the neck.*

Modalities for diagnosis
- Duplex ultrasound.
- MRI to establish the extent.
- Lymphoscintigraphy to assess lymphedema and draining vessels.
- Biopsy for microcystic lesions to differentiate from other skin lesions.
- Genetic studies.

Treatment
- Compression stockings, prevention of infection or trauma.
- Extratruncular lesions – treated with irritant sclerosants such as doxycycline, bleomycin, ethanol or sodium tetradecylsulfate.
- Large circumscribed lesions (cystic hygroma) may be surgically excised.
- Truncular LMs are managed as for lymphedema.

Capillary malformations
- These used to be called 'port-wine stains'.
- They can occur independently or in combination with other CVMs.
- Duplex ultrasound may be used to rule out an underlying VM or AVM.
- Treatment is mostly for cosmetic reasons.
- The main form of treatment is vascular laser therapy.

Arteriovenous malformations (Fig. 12.5)
Presentation
- This is the most aggressive form of CVM.
- An active extratruncular AVM allows arteriovenous shunting with high flow due to absence of restriction at a capillary level, as well as retaining a nidus (central area of direct AV connections) capable of rapid multiplication and a high rate of recurrence (Fig. 12.6).

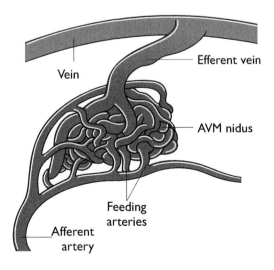

Fig. 12.5 *Clinical appearance of an AVM of the lumbar region.*

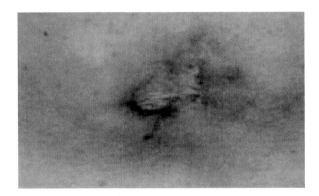

Fig. 12.6 *Arteriovenous malformation.*
- *Abnormal vessels connect an artery and a vein.*

- Initially presents with localized swelling, thrill and a bruit.
- Later presents with features of arterial 'steal syndrome' ranging from cutaneous blanching in a reticulate pattern, ulceration, and gangrene to skin necrosis.
- Larger AVMs can result in cardiac failure.
- Truncular AVMs are extremely rare. They allow a direct communication between an artery and a vein with no nidus.
- Truncular AVMs include pulmonary AVF and patent ductus arteriosus.
- *Parkes Weber syndrome** consists of a truncular AVM in association with the following (Fig. 12.7):
  - Cutaneous capillary malformations (portwine stain).
  - Venous and lymphatic malformations.
  - Skeletal or soft-tissue hypertrophy.
  - Overgrowth of one limb, usually the leg.

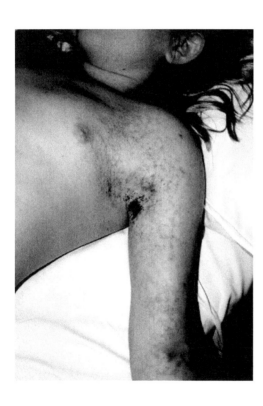

Fig. 12.7 *Clinical appearance of a lesion associated with Parkes Weber syndrome.*

Modalities for diagnosis
- Baseline evaluation is with:
  - Duplex ultrasound.
  - Whole-body blood pool scintigraphy (WBBPS).
  - Transarterial lung perfusion scintigraphy (TLPS).
  - MRI.
  - MR angiography (MRA).
  - MRV.
  - Computed tomography (CT).

*Frederick Parkes Weber, 1863–1962, English dermatologist

- Confirmation of final diagnosis should be made with:
  - Selective and superselective arteriography.
  - Direct puncture arteriography.
  - Standard and/or direct puncture venography.

Indications for treatment
Absolute
- Hemorrhage.
- High-output heart failure.
- Secondary arterial ischemia.
- Secondary complications from chronic venous hypertension.
- Lesions located at a life-threatening region such as adjacent to the airway, at a region threatening vital functions such as vision, or in a region with a potentially high risk of complications such as hemarthrosis.

Relative
- Disabling pain.
- Severe functional impairment.
- Cosmetically severe deformity.
- High risk of complications.

Treatment
- There are different management strategies for different types of CVMs.
- It is essential to assess the extent, severity, and progression before treatment.
- It is best to manage a dormant CVM expectantly.
- Early aggressive treatment may be required to prevent life- or limb-threatening complications.
- It is essential to ensure that the benefits from intervention exceed morbidity from treatment because ill-planned intervention can stimulate explosive growth.
- Simply closing the feeding artery leaving the nidus intact usually makes the condition worse by provoking more aggressive neovascular growth. The nidus must be controlled to prevent recurrence.
- However, it is rarely possible to completely eradicate the nidus due to excessive tissue destruction from chemical ablation or excessive bleeding from surgery.
- Coil embolization of the enlarged high-flow efferent vein is the most effective means to reduce flow rates allowing the nidus to be more readily treated by sclerotherapy or in some cases by surgical excision.
- Complications of treatment include arterial embolization, tissue destruction by sclerosant, severe swelling with progression to compartment syndrome, pulmonary embolism (PE) and end-organ ischemia.

CLINICAL ASPECTS – ACQUIRED AVF
- An AVF is an abnormal connection between an artery and a vein.
- Acquired AVF results from trauma or disease.
- AVFs can affect any site in the body.
- Some are inaccessible to ultrasound examination such as cerebral, spinal cord, pulmonary or coronary AVFs.

- However, AVFs affecting the extremities or viscera are well suited to detection and assessment by ultrasound.
- Angiography is usually required before treatment.

Etiology
Trauma
- Accidental from blunt or penetrating trauma.
- Iatrogenic from needle biopsy, arterial puncture or intravenous catheter insertion.

Disease
- Neoplasia such as renal carcinoma.
- Aneurysms such as rupture of an abdominal aortic aneurysm into the inferior vena cava.

Clinical features
- Pulsatile swelling if superficial.
- Machinery murmur with auscultation.
- Reduced pulse rate with digital occlusion of the AVF.

Complications
- High-pressure arterial flow entering veins through an AVF in the limbs leading to thin-walled varicosities.
- Bleeding such as with hematuria from a renal AVF.
- Reduced distal perfusion causing ischemia from a large AVF.
- High-output heart failure from a large AVF.

Treatment
- Surgical separation and repair of the associated vessels.
- Endovascular placement of an intra-arterial stent-graft.
- Endovascular coil embolization.

WHAT DOCTORS NEED TO KNOW

- Is the lesion a hemangioma, CVM or acquired AVF?
- Do flow characteristics allow classification of a CVM?
- What is its extent and depth and does it extend into deeper muscle or bone?

THE DUPLEX SCAN

Abbreviations
- Peak systolic velocity (cm/s) – PSV.

Indications for scanning
- To establish the diagnosis.
- To help assess the extent and depth.
- Serial scans to assess the natural history or response to treatment.

NOTE!

- Always take a clinical history.
- A CVM is present at birth whereas HOIs appear later.
- A CVM will grow proportionate to the child's growth whereas HOIs grow rapidly.
- A HOI can be confused with an AVM in children.
- A NICH can be confused with an AVM in adults.
- Hemangiomas present as a soft-tissue mass whereas an AVM is highly vascular.

Ultrasound findings

Hemangioma

- B-mode shows a discrete solid mass with low internal echogenicity (Fig. 12.8a).
- When the lesion is active, color and spectral Doppler demonstrate intralesional flow with mean PSV of approximately 12 cm/s (Fig. 12.8b).
- When the lesion is involuted, minimal flow is demonstrated on color and spectral Doppler.

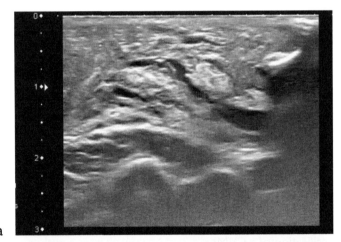

a

b

Fig. 12.8 *Ultrasound images of a HOI:*
a *B-mode.*
b *Color and spectral Doppler.*

Venous malformation
- On B-mode, a patent extratruncular VM is a compressible lesion (Fig. 12.9) with low flow rates on spectral Doppler.

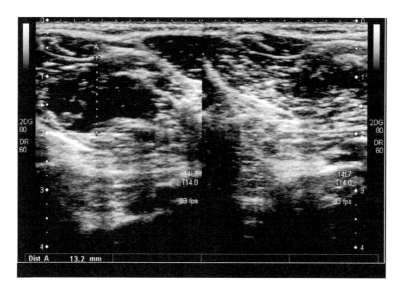

Fig. 12.9 *B-mode image demonstrating compressibility of a VM.*

Lymphatic malformation
- On B-mode an extratruncular LM is an incompressible lesion with thin walls (Fig. 12.10) and no flow on color or spectral Doppler within the lesion.

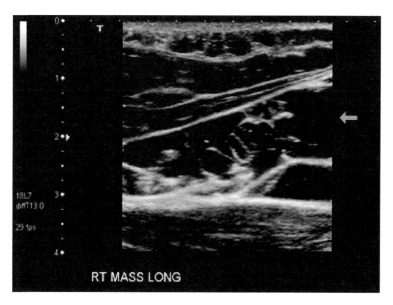

Fig. 12.10 *B-mode image of an LM.*
- *Note the lymphatic cysts.*

Arteriovenous malformation

- On B-mode, an AVM is an incompressible lesion (Fig. 12.11a) with highly pulsatile flow on spectral Doppler.
- If a nidus is present, color Doppler will demonstrate turbulent flow and aliasing within the nidus (Fig. 12.11b).
- Dilated, thickened, tortuous associated vessels on B-mode.
- Spectral Doppler will demonstrate arterialized flow in the associated veins with medial thickening and fibrosis on B-mode.

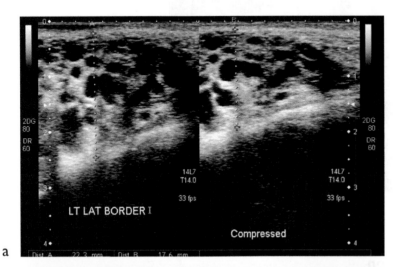

a

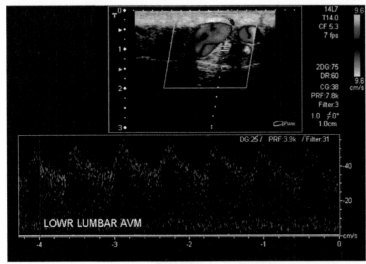

b

Fig. 12.11 *Ultrasound images of an AVM:*
a *B-mode image of incompressibility.*
b *Color and spectral Doppler of the nidus.*

Successfully treated CVMs

- When fully thrombosed these lesions will demonstrate no flow on color, power and spectral Doppler.

Acquired AVFs

- Spectral Doppler demonstrates low-resistance flow in the afferent artery.
- Spectral Doppler demonstrates a turbulent high-velocity flow signal in the AVF (Fig. 12.12).
- Spectral Doppler demonstrates a high-velocity arterialized waveform in the efferent vein.

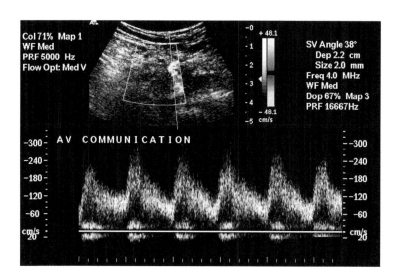

Fig. 12.12 *Spectral Doppler trace from an AVF.*

PROTOCOLS FOR SCANNING

Select transducer

- A high frequency linear transducer is suitable.

TIP!

- Always compare with the contralateral side to establish the normal anatomy and normal flow characteristics.

Scan with B-mode

- Determine if the lesion is compressible and whether it contains thrombus.
- Measure the width, depth and length.
- Detect deeper involvement of underlying muscle and other tissues.
- Measure location from an anatomical landmark.
- Relate the lesion to adjacent normal arteries and veins.
- Measure the size and number of lymphatic cysts for LM.
- Scan for evidence of soft-tissue or bone hypertrophy.
- Detect occlusion from treatment using B-mode to test for compressibility and measure the size of the lesion.

Scan with color and spectral Doppler

- Determine whether the lesion is predominantly soft tissue (hemangioma) or predominantly vascular channels with little soft tissue (CVM).

- Determine flow characteristics of high, low or no flow.
- Determine if flow is continuous or low-resistance pulsatile.
- Record sample spectral traces within the associated veins, arteries and nidus (if present), and record mean PSV.
- Detect occlusion from treatment using color and spectral Doppler to interrogate for patency.

ULTRASOUND IMAGES TO RECORD

Pre-treatment

- B-mode image of lesion.
- B-mode measurements of width, length, and depth of lesion.
- Note location of lesion from an anatomical landmark.
- Note relationship to adjacent veins and arteries.
- Note soft-tissue or bone hypertrophy.
- Note size and number of lymphatic cysts in LMs.
- B-mode in transverse dual image of lesion not compressed and compressed.
- Color Doppler image of lesion.
- Spectral traces in afferent arteries, efferent veins, and nidus; note mean PSVs and waveform morphology.
- Comparative images from the contralateral side.

Post-treatment

- B-mode image of lesion.
- B-mode measurements of width, length, and depth of lesion.
- B-mode in transverse dual image of lesion not compressed and compressed.
- Color Doppler image of lesion.
- Sample spectral traces in associated vessels and nidus.

WORKSHEET

- Draw a diagram representing the type of lesion and its location with appropriate B-mode measurement, flow velocities and waveform morphology.

13 HEMODIALYSIS STUDIES

Chronic renal failure is usually irreversible. It can be treated by hemodialysis after surgical formation of an arteriovenous direct anastomosis or interposition vein graft to form an arteriovenous fistula (AVF) or arteriovenous synthetic graft (AVG). An alternate technique is peritoneal dialysis. Acute renal failure is frequently reversible and is usually treated by hemodialysis through a central venous catheter. However, this is not suitable for long-term treatment due to a limited lifespan. Ultrasound is used to assess suitability of upper limb vessels for AVF or AVG placement, follow maturation of an AVF and detect complications of an AVF or AVG that might lead to access failure.

ANATOMY

Vessels scanned for reporting:
- Internal jugular vein – IJV
- Innominate artery and veins
- Subclavian artery and vein
- Axillary artery and vein
- Brachial artery and veins
- Radial artery and veins
- Ulnar artery and veins
- Basilic and cephalic veins
- Deep and superficial arterial and venous palmar arches.

PRINCIPLES OF HEMODIALYSIS

- Surgery is performed to create a connection between an artery and a vein.
- This can be by direct anastomosis or interposition vein graft (AVF) or synthetic graft (AVG).
- Long-term patency requires an adequate inflow and outflow.
- Treatment is usually performed three times a week and each session usually lasts for 3–4 hours.
- An AVF is superior to an AVG because it is far less prone to complications including thrombosis and infection and has better long-term patency rates. It should be possible to place an AVF in most patients even after multiple prior procedures.
- However, an AVG can be used within about 2 weeks whereas an AVF takes some 6 weeks to 'mature' before it can be used.
- There is an immediate four- to fivefold increase in venous flow in an AVF or AVG and up to a tenfold increase in an AVF within a few weeks.
- At least 20% of AVFs fail to mature sufficiently to allow hemodialysis.
- A flow volume of 200–400 ml/min is required for satisfactory dialysis.
- A flow volume >15–20% of cardiac output could lead to high-output heart failure.
- Dialysis is continued until a kidney transplantation has been performed.

- A schematic representation of hemodialysis is shown in Fig. 13.1:
  - A large-bore needle at the proximal end of the vein withdraws blood. This is then pumped through the hemodialysis machine.
  - This filters blood through a semipermeable membrane to remove toxic chemicals such as urea and creatinine which are normally excreted by the kidneys.
  - Purified blood is then returned through another large-bore needle placed in the distal end of the vein.

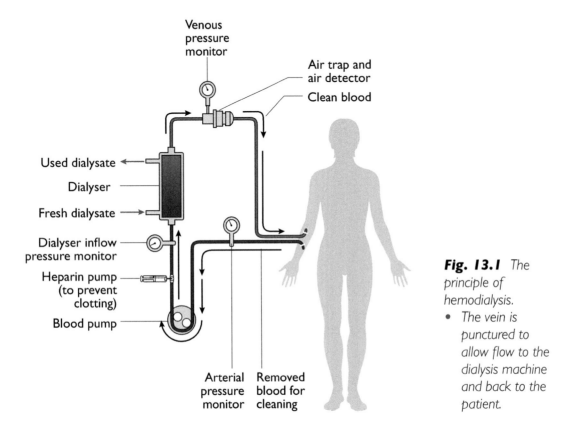

Fig. 13.1 *The principle of hemodialysis.*
- *The vein is punctured to allow flow to the dialysis machine and back to the patient.*

Techniques for an AVF or AVG

- An AVF can be performed by direct anastomosis at any site where the artery and vein are relatively close together. This is most often a radiocephalic AVF at the wrist (Brescia–Cimino* AVF) (Fig. 13.2) or brachiobasilic or brachiocephalic AVF at the cubital fossa (Fig. 13.3).
- Direct anastomosis may be side-to-side, end-to-side, or end-to-end (Fig. 13.4).
- Alternately, an AVF can be formed by anastomosing a loop of transposed saphenous vein graft if the artery and vein are a distance apart.
- A synthetic AVG can be formed, usually with a length of a 5–6 mm diameter polytetrafluoroethylene (PTFE) graft in either the arm (Fig. 13.5) or the leg (Fig. 13.6).
- If all other options have been exhausted, it is possible to remove the femoral vein and a short segment of great saphenous vein from the leg, and anastomose the two to form a composite interposition graft in the arm. The femoral vein is a large-caliber vein for cannulation and the great saphenous vein has sufficient resistance to flow to prevent cardiac failure.

---

*M Brescia and J Cimino – surgeons from New York who described the technique in 1966

- An AVF consists of several segments:
  - ○ Afferent (carry to) inflow artery.
  - ○ Arteriovenous anastomosis.
  - ○ Swing site (mobilized segment).
  - ○ Segment of efferent (carry away) vein for needling.
  - ○ Central veins.
- The segment of vein for needling is ideally about 10 cm long and it should be at least 6 cm long. If the two needles are too close, unpurified and purified blood will mix, resulting in less efficient dialysis.

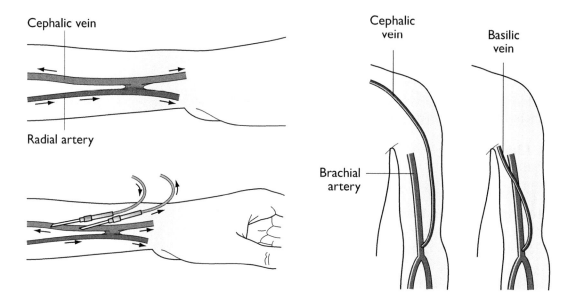

Fig. 13.2 *Side-to-side AVF at the wrist.*
- *The preferred technique is to anastomose the cephalic vein to the radial artery.*

Fig. 13.3 *End-to-side AVF at the cubital fossa.*
- *Anastomosis can be to the cephalic or basilic vein.*

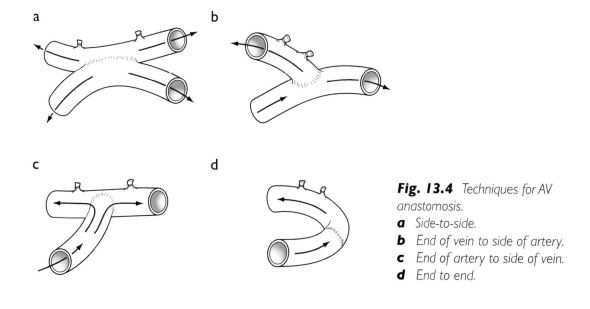

Fig. 13.4 *Techniques for AV anastomosis.*
- *a Side-to-side.*
- *b End of vein to side of artery.*
- *c End of artery to side of vein.*
- *d End to end.*

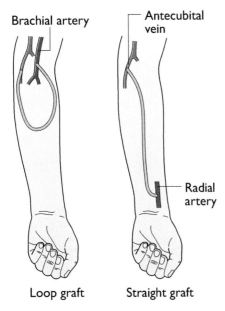

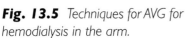

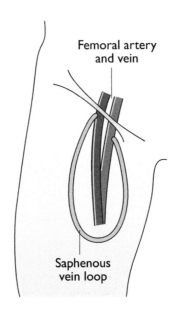

Fig. 13.5 *Techniques for AVG for hemodialysis in the arm.*

Fig. 13.6 *A technique for AVG for hemodialysis in the leg.*

Selection for the best site for an AVF or AVG

- Selection of the best artery and vein to provide access is crucial to obtaining the best long-term patency rates.
- An AVF or AVG is most often formed in the non-dominant arm. However, it can be performed in the dominant arm or leg if the anatomy in the non-dominant arm is unsuitable, particularly after past failed procedures.
- It is best to form an AVF or AVG in the right arm if a pacemaker is present.
- Prior central venous catheter placement can cause thrombosis in the upper limb veins.
- For older or diabetic patients with peripheral arterial disease, it is best to fashion the AVF or AVG at a more proximal level away from the site of arterial disease.
- Preoperative ultrasound assessment for arterial disease is very helpful to determine the best site for the AV shunt.
- Younger patients with normal peripheral arteries should have an AVF constructed distally to allow subsequent access to more proximal vessels if repeat surgery is required.

AVF and AVG maturation

- The intention is to 'mature' the vein to increase its diameter and wall thickness over a sufficient length to allow it to be used for hemodialysis.
- Maturation of an AVF takes approximately 6 weeks to allow it to become large and thick enough to allow repeated needling which provides an adequate flow rate to the hemodialysis machine.
- There are several reasons why the vein may not mature or function well:
  - There are large vein tributaries.
  - A perforating vein steals flow from the superficial vein.
  - Venous outflow is inadequate.
  - The vein is too deep to cannulate.
- An AVG can be used for dialysis approximately 2 weeks after placement.

Complications

- Thrombosis from repeated cannulations causing obstructed outflow is the most common complication for a synthetic AVG.
- Thrombosis may also occur due to selection of inadequately sized arteries and veins for AVF or AVG placement, or may be caused by external compression by hematoma or fluid collection.
- Anastomotic stenosis may occur due to neointimal hyperplasia and also from kinking, twisting, hypoplasia or atherosclerotic plaque and this is the most common complication for an AVF. Anastomotic stenosis is most common at the venous end.
- Hematoma or false aneurysm can result from needling or infection.
- True aneurysm can occur due to degradation of the AVG wall.
- Perigraft fluid collection can occur.
- Infection is most common in a groin AVG.
- Steal of arterial flow from the hand can occur (Fig. 13.7). Flow will be away from the hand through the distal radial artery.
- Excessive shunt flow can cause high-output cardiac failure.
- Venous anastomosis is the most common site for stenosis with a groin AVG.

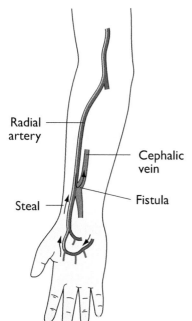

Radial artery

Cephalic vein

Steal

Fistula

Fig. 13.7 *AVF steal.*

Clinical presentation of complications

- The following clinical features suggest that an AVF or AVG is failing, stenosed or occluded:
  - Failure of vein to dilate or mature.
  - Elevation of venous pressure.
  - Swelling of the arm with superficial collateral veins.
  - Poor flow for dialysis.
  - Reduction or absence of the normal palpable 'thrill'.
  - Slow clotting after dialysis.
  - Increased arterial pump pressure.

- A steal from the circulation to the hand is manifest by the following features:
  - Pain in the hand or fingers.
  - Ischemic necrosis.
- Palpable aneurysm.

Indications for location of stenosis causing complications

- Afferent artery stenosis:
  - Steal from the hand.
- Swing segment stenosis:
  - Inability to reach adequate pump speed on dialysis machine.
  - Increased arterial pump pressure.
  - Failure of AVF to mature.
  - Reduction or absence of 'thrill'.
- Venous outflow stenosis:
  - Elevation of venous pressure.
  - Slow clotting after dialysis.
- Chronic venous outflow thrombosis:
  - Swollen arm with superficial collateral veins.

Treatment of complications

- Approximately one-third of asymptomatic patients have an abnormality in an AVF or AVG shown by ultrasound. Initially, this may simply warrant observation rather than immediate intervention.
- However, early detection of a failing AVF or AVG by ultrasound allows the decision to intervene before it occludes.
- The decision to intervene is based on a significant reduction in flow volume rather than detection of a high-grade stenosis.
- Stenosis or thrombosis of an AVF or AVG may require surgical revision, percutaneous balloon dilatation or percutaneous thrombolysis.
- True aneurysms may remain stable for years and do not necessarily require treatment if the overlying skin is intact.
- False aneurysms <5 mm in diameter are often not clinically significant but if they are >5 mm in diameter they have a tendency to enlarge and should be treated by embolization or surgical repair.

WHAT DOCTORS NEED TO KNOW

- Are the arterial and venous systems suitable for construction of an AVF or AVG?
- Can a fistula be formed or is a graft necessary?
- Where is the best site for the AVF or AVG?
- Is the vein maturing to allow hemodialysis?
- Is the AVF or AVG remaining free from complications?

THE DUPLEX SCAN

Abbreviations
- Peak systolic velocity (cm/s) – PSV
- Volume flow (ml/min) – VF = cross-sectional area (cm^2) × mean velocity (cm/s) × 60.

Volume flow
- This is measured in arteries because they have a circular cross-section, enabling an accurate area to be obtained from the inner lumen diameter.
- Volume flow measurements from veins can be erroneous due to non-circular cross-section and non-axial flow.
- Ultrasound machines can calculate cross-sectional area from a diameter measurement and the mean velocity from spectral waveforms over a few cardiac cycles.
- Volume flow should be measured in either the subclavian or the brachial arteries even for a wrist AVF or AVG because most of the flow from these arteries goes to the AVF or AVG.
- Spectral sample volume should encompass the entire vessel lumen to gain an accurate mean velocity.

Indications for scanning
- Assessment for suitability of arteries and veins for an AVF or AVG.
- Assessment of the effect on the circulation to the hand before constructing an AVF or AVG.
- Serial studies for maturation of an AVF.
- Investigation for loss of the palpable thrill.
- Investigation for insufficient flow for hemodialysis.
- Failure to mature AVF.
- Investigation for inability to cannulate for hemodialysis.
- Investigation of slow clotting after decannulation.
- Serial studies to detect complications in an AVF or AVG.
- Monitoring of known AVF or AVG stenosis.

Normal findings
Selection of vessels suitable for an AVF or AVG
- Normal arteries with triphasic flow continuous from the major branches of the aortic arch to the wrist.
- No stenosis or occlusion in upper limb arteries (see Chapter 5).
- Phasicity with respiration and pulsatility in proximal arm veins.
- Continuous venous outflow pathway >2 mm diameter.
- No venous thrombosis or wall thickening.
- The vein is accessible for cannulation.

Definition of a mature AVF
- Efferent vein diameter >5 mm over a length >6 cm.

Features of a normal functioning AVF or AVG

- High-velocity, low-resistance waveform in the afferent artery.
- Pulsatile flow in the efferent vein.
- Sudden changes in direction of flow in an AVF.
- High PSV of up to 350 cm/s in the AVF or AVG (Fig. 13.8) causing a palpable thrill and high-frequency bruit indicating turbulence.
- Volume flow from 300 ml/min to 1200 ml/min to the hemodialysis machine.
- Wall thickening of the vein adjacent to the AVF or AVG anastomosis.
- Non-axial turbulent flow in veins close to the anastomosis.
- Veins that normally demonstrate pulsatile and phasic flow to the level of the axillary or even the subclavian vein.
- Needling segment of vein <10 mm deep to skin surface for an ideal length of ≥8 cm.

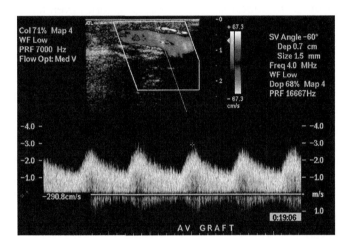

Fig. 13.8 A spectral tracing at the anastomosis of a normally functioning AVF for hemodialysis.

Criteria for AVF or AVG stenosis (Fig 13.9)

- B-mode showing AVF lumen diameter <3 mm; this might be larger in a proximal fistula in a large male than a distal fistula in a small female.
- Volume flow <300 ml/min for AVF or <600 ml/s for AVG.

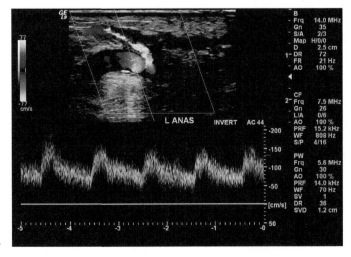

a

Fig. 13.9 AVF stenosis:
a Spectral Doppler trace in afferent artery just proximal to AVF.

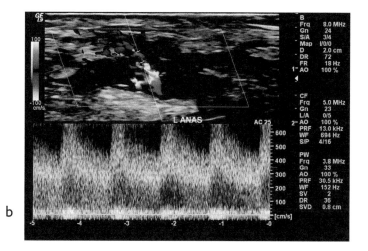

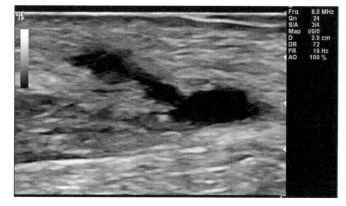

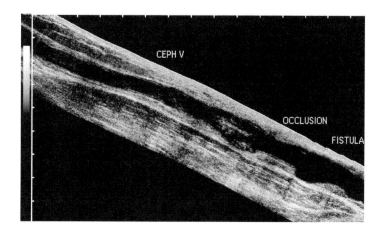

Fig. 13.9 (continued)
b Spectral Doppler trace in AVF stenosis.
c B-mode image of AVF stenosis.

Images kindly supplied by Martin Necas, Hamilton, New Zealand.

- Return to high-resistance flow in the afferent artery.
- PSV >400 cm/s or sudden increase in PSV ratio to 3:1 in the AVF or afferent artery.
- PSV <150 cm/s in the efferent vein.
- Post-stenotic turbulence in the efferent vein.

Criteria for AVF or AVG occlusion

- Absence of flow with spectral and color Doppler and possible visualization of echogenic material filling the vessel lumen in the afferent artery, efferent vein (Fig. 13.10) or AVG

Fig. 13.10 B-mode image of echogenic material filling the efferent vein due to occlusion.

Image kindly supplied by Martin Necas, Hamilton, New Zealand.

- Return to high-resistance usually triphasic flow in the afferent artery
- Refer to previous volume flow criteria.

Criteria for hand 'steal'
- Reversed flow in the artery distal to the AVF or AVG.
- Compensatory increased flow in the saved forearm artery.
- Volume flow >1600 ml/min can indicate the potential for hand 'steal'.

Criteria for aneurysm
- Diameter increased by more than twice the preceding diameter.
- Diameter increased >15 mm.
- A false aneurysm will appear as a localized outpouching with flow on color Doppler (Fig. 13.11).

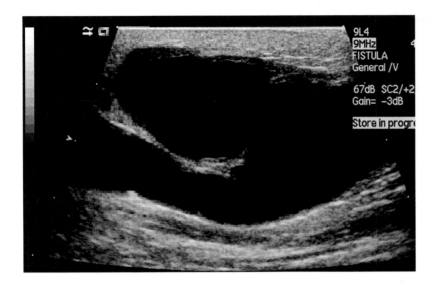

Fig. 13.11 *B-mode image of false aneurysm.*

Image kindly supplied by Martin Necas, Hamilton, New Zealand.

PROTOCOLS FOR SCANNING

- Preparing the patient, selecting the best transducer, and general principles for scanning are discussed in Chapter 3 (pages 39–40).

Position the patient and select windows
- Examine the IJV with the patient supine to distend the vein walls.
- For proximal vessels, examine the patient seated or standing so that the shoulder girdle is relaxed and falls down under gravity to improve access.
- Examine subclavian and axillary vessels through suprasternal, supraclavicular and infraclavicular windows.
- Use copious gel to maintain good skin contact in the suprasternal notch and over superficial aneurysms.
- The axillary artery is easier to see with the arm abducted and scanned from an axillary approach, but it can be scanned through an anterior window.
- With the patient upright or lying supine, externally rotate the arm to view the brachial vessels from a medial window between triceps and biceps.

- It may be easier to scan with the patient supine and the arm externally rotated for the vessels of the forearm, or examine with the patient sitting and the arm resting on a support with the palm rotated upwards.
- If an AVG is in the groin, lay the patient supine with the appropriate leg rotated outwards.

Optimize the image

- There is a trade-off between a high-frequency linear transducer for good spatial resolution and a lower-frequency linear transducer with a higher pulse repetition frequency (PRF) which is therefore less prone to aliasing with high velocities in the AVF or AVG.
- Reduce color gain to attempt to reduce vibration artifacts caused by the 'thrill' which can obscure vessel interrogation.
- The vibration artifact may be reduced by compressing the patient's arm adjacent to the transducer with the sonographer's hand, making sure to avoid compressing the vein.
- Open the spectral sample volume to cover the entire width of the vessels. Mean velocities will be overestimated if the sample volume covers only the center of the vessels.
- Set the color and spectral scale high to minimize color Doppler aliasing in the high-flow circulation.

Scan to assess suitability for an AVF or AVG

- Use spectral Doppler to test for phasicity and pulsatility in the innominate and subclavian veins and the IJV.
- Use color and spectral Doppler with distal augmentation and compression testing in B-mode to determine patency of all deep and superficial upper limb veins distal to clavicle.
- Use B-mode to identify thrombus in any veins and measure location from an anatomical landmark and the extent.
- Note the level of any tributaries and perforators that communicate with the cephalic or basilic veins and measure their level from the elbow crease. Ensure that the cephalic and basilic veins are superficial at all levels.
- In transverse B-mode, measure lumen diameters of the cephalic and basilic veins noting location and extent from the elbow crease of any segment of diameter <2 mm.
- Use color and spectral Doppler to ensure the patency of all upper limb arteries and to classify the degree of stenosis (see Chapter 5). Use B-mode to classify the plaque type (see Chapter 6).
- Note the level of the brachial artery bifurcation from an anatomical landmark.
- Note the level of the basilic vein entering the brachial vein to ensure a long enough segment to be 'swung' around.
- Note anatomical variations.

Scan to examine an AVF or AVG

- If possible, study on a day when there are no dressings applied.
- Use B-mode in transverse to measure native vessel lumen diameter and the AVG or AVF diameters.
- Use color and spectral Doppler to determine flow directions and detect stenosis or occlusion.
- Commence examination in the subclavian artery and scan through the brachial artery.
- In either the subclavian or the brachial artery in longitudinal, take a sample spectral trace to determine mean velocity and in B-mode in transverse measure the lumen diameter to calculate VF. Repeat three times to calculate an average VF measurement.

- 'Walk' the spectral sample volume through the afferent artery to the AVG arterial anastomosis or the AVF, investigating for stenosis or occlusion. Adjust the cursor angle as you 'walk' the sample volume through the connection to the efferent vein.
- Take sample spectral traces within the anastomosis and swing sites of the AVF.
- Take sample spectral traces within both anastomosis sites and the mid-AVG.
- Take spectral traces proximal to, at and distal to stenosis. Note the location from an anatomical landmark and the extent.
- Take a spectral trace to demonstrate occlusion by thrombosis. Note the location from an anatomical landmark and the extent.
- Determine the age of the thrombus (Chapter 10, pages 187–188) and whether fully or partially occlusive (Fig. 13.12).
- Take a sample spectral trace from the artery distal to the anastomosis to determine flow direction and detect steal from the hand.
- Take a sample spectral trace in the efferent vein, and in transverse B-mode measure the lumen diameter.
- With color and spectral Doppler, determine if the flow is directed away from the efferent vein through unexpected venous pathways. Describe the location of these veins.
- Note if aneurysms are present and measure proximal, maximum and distal diameters in transverse B-mode. Measure the length of an aneurysm and location from an anatomical landmark.
- For false aneurysms, measure their maximum diameter and the diameter and length of the neck. Note the location from an anatomical landmark.
- Note if mural thrombus is present in any aneurysms and measure the residual lumen diameter.
- Note the presence of any collections. Use color Doppler to differentiate from an aneurysm.
- If needling is difficult, in B-mode measure the depth of the efferent vein from the surface of the skin.

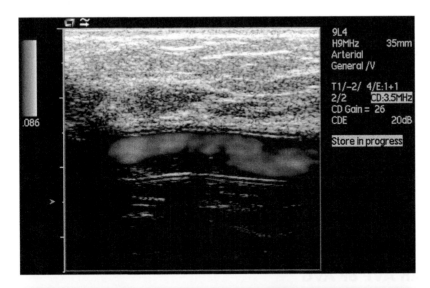

Fig. 13.12 *Power Doppler image of partially occlusive thrombus in an AVG.*

Image kindly supplied by Martin Necas, Hamilton, New Zealand.

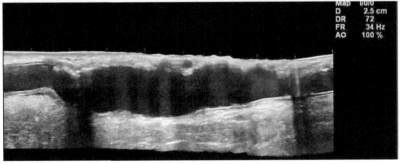

Fig. 13.13 *B-mode image of efferent vein wall damage due to frequent needling.*

Image kindly supplied by Martin Necas, Hamilton, New Zealand.

- Scan for damage to the efferent vein wall due to frequent needling (Fig. 13.13).
- Continue scanning up the arm to the proximal veins, including the IJV.
- Measure the length and note the location relative to the elbow crease of any segment of the efferent vein <5 mm diameter.

TIPS!

- Hold the probe in transverse to identify the full course of the AVF or AVG from the afferent artery to the efferent vein.
- Interrogate vessels in longitudinal to record spectral traces.
- Use very light pressure with the transducer so as not to compress the superficial veins in the pre-AVF or -AVG assessment. The postoperative efferent vein may be more difficult to erroneously compress due to its increased pressure.
- If possible, select a lower-frequency transducer if too much aliasing is a problem.

PITFALLS!

- Shadowing from excessive scar tissue or calcification may obscure full insonation of an AVG.
- Color bruits may obscure color flow in an AVF or AVG stenosis.

ULTRASOUND IMAGES TO RECORD

Preoperative assessment of AVF or AVG

Veins

- Sample spectral trace in longitudinal for flow in the proximal veins with normal respiration and the Valsalva maneuver.
- B-mode in longitudinal of the subclavian artery during a sniff test.
- Transverse B-mode dual images to demonstrate compressibility of all superficial and deep veins of the arm.
- Sample spectral trace of all mid- to distal veins during distal augmentation.
- Spectral trace and color Doppler images to demonstrate lack of flow in thrombosed veins.
- Note location of thrombus from an anatomical landmark and extent.
- Transverse B-mode images of the lumen diameters of cephalic and basilic veins, noting. distance from an anatomical landmark if diameter is <2 mm.

Arteries

- Sample spectral traces in longitudinal for all arteries listed.
- Spectral traces proximal to, at and distal to each stenosis; note the location from an anatomical landmark, the extent, and the severity.
- B-mode of plaques in longitudinal.

- Spectral traces proximal to, distal to and within occlusions; note the location from an anatomical landmark and the extent.
- Transverse B-mode image of the lumen diameter of all arteries listed, noting distance from an anatomical landmark if diameter <2 mm.
- Note level of brachial artery bifurcation from the elbow crease.

Postoperative assessment of AVF or AVG

- Sample spectral traces for all arteries and veins listed; note the flow direction and waveform morphology.
- Sample spectral trace in artery distal to AVF or AVG; note the flow direction.
- Transverse B-mode images of the lumen diameters for all arteries and veins listed.
- Three VF measurements from either the brachial or the subclavian artery.
- Transverse B-mode images of the lumen diameters of AVF, mid-AVG and anastomosis sites.
- Sample spectral traces in AVF, mid-AVG and anastomosis sites.
- Spectral traces proximal to, at and distal to stenosis; note the location from an anatomical landmark and severity.
- Spectral traces proximal to, distal to and within occlusions; note the location from an anatomical landmark and the extent.
- B-mode of the length of an aneurysm in longitudinal.
- B-mode of maximum transverse and anteroposterior diameters of an aneurysm.
- B-mode of length and diameter of neck of a false aneurysm.
- B-mode of mural thrombus and residual lumen diameter of an aneurysm.
- B-mode of proximal and distal diameters of vessel adjacent to an aneurysm.

WORKSHEET

- Draw a diagram representing the location of AVF or AVG with appropriate diameters, velocities, VF measurements and stenosis or occlusion locations recorded.

MALE GENITAL VASCULAR DISORDERS

Duplex scanning can be used to study erectile dysfunction in males because it is relatively atraumatic and inexpensive. It helps to establish the cause to enable better choice of appropriate treatment. However, ultrasound is less widely used now since the introduction of sildenafil citrate (Viagra) and other similar drugs which are used to treat all causes. Ultrasound is widely used to diagnose acute conditions affecting the testis and associated structures, as well as to diagnose varicocele.

ANATOMY

Vessels scanned for reporting:
- Aorta
- Common iliac artery – CIA
- Internal iliac artery – IIA
- Common penile artery
- Cavernosal artery
- Testicular (internal spermatic) artery and vein
- Pampiniform vein plexus.

Other vessels discussed:
- Internal pudendal artery and vein
- Bulbourethral artery
- Dorsal artery
- Circumflex artery
- Helicine arteries
- Superficial dorsal vein
- Deep dorsal vein
- Deferential artery
- Cremasteric artery
- Left renal vein
- Internal iliac vein – IIV
- Inferior vena cava – IVC
- Superficial external pudendal artery and vein
- Common femoral artery – CFA.

Penis (Fig. 14.1)
- The penis consists of three parallel cylinders:
  - Paired corpora cavernosa.
  - A single corpus spongiosum.
- The corpora cavernosa form the main part of the body and contain erectile tissue.
- They are located dorsolateral separated by an incomplete median septum.
- At the base of the penis the septum is more complete.
- The corpora cavernosa and corpus spongiosum are surrounded by the tunica albuginea, a dense fibrous sheath of connective tissue with relatively few elastic fibers.

- The tunica albuginea surrounding the corpus spongiosum is thinner and more elastic to allow for distension and passage of ejaculate through the urethra.
- Superficial to the tunica albuginea is the deep penile (Buck's) fascia. Buck's fascia constrains the deep dorsal vein preventing venous return and sustaining erection.

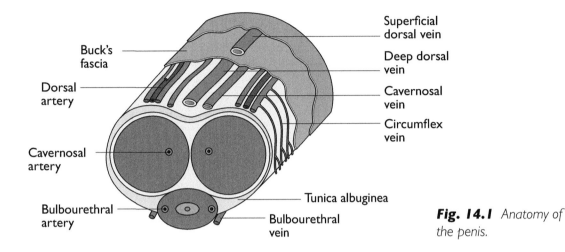

Fig. 14.1 *Anatomy of the penis.*

Penile arterial supply (Figs 14.1 and 14.2)

- The arterial supply to the penis is from the IIAs.
- The internal pudendal artery is a branch of the IIA and continues as the common penile artery.
- The common penile artery divides into three paired right and left branches:
  - The bulbourethral arteries supply the corpus spongiosum and the urethra.
  - The cavernosal arteries supply the corpus cavernosum.
  - The dorsal arteries supply the skin and glans penis.
- The cavernosal arteries give off small branches termed 'helicine arteries' which are integral in the erectile process.
- The blood supply to the skin of the penis is from the right and left superficial external pudendal arteries which are a branch of the CFA.

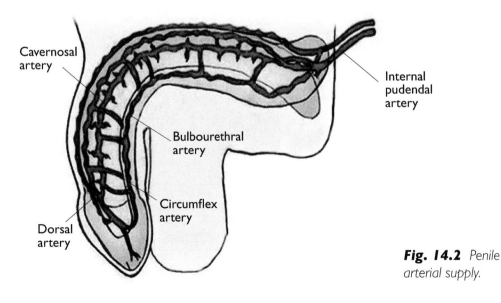

Fig. 14.2 *Penile arterial supply.*

Penile venous drainage (Figs 14.1 and 14.3)

- The superficial dorsal vein lies superficial to Buck's fascia and drains through the superficial external pudendal veins to the saphenofemoral junction.
- The deep dorsal vein lies within Buck's fascia and drains mainly through the pudendal plexus to the IIVs.
- The deep dorsal vein takes blood from the corpus cavernosum through the circumflex and emissary veins.

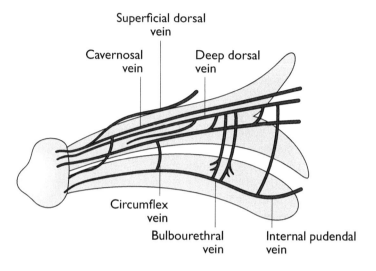

Fig. 14.3 *Penile venous drainage.*

Scrotum, testes and appendages (Fig. 14.4)

- The scrotum has two compartments, each containing a testis, epididymis, and spermatic cord.
- The tunica albuginea is a fibrous layer that contains the testis.
- The tunica vaginalis is a serous layer that contains the testis and tunica albuginea.
- Normally, the tunica vaginalis attaches posteriorly to the scrotum and epididymis so as to anchor the testis.

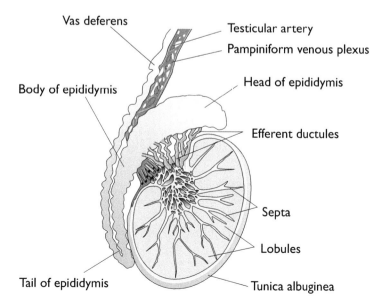

Fig. 14.4 *Anatomy of intrascrotal structures.*

- The tunica vaginalis has a visceral and parietal lamina with a small amount of fluid between the layers.
- The mediastinum testis is a network of fibrous tissue that extends craniocaudal through the testis.
- Septa are given off from the mediastinum and attach to the tunica albuginea. The septa divide the testis into lobules and these contain the seminiferous tubules which converge to the epididymis.
- The epididymis lies along the posterolateral aspect of the testis and is where sperm are matured and stored.
- The epididymis consists of a head at the upper end, a body and a tail at the lower end.
- The tail becomes the vas deferens which ascends out of the scrotum.
- The spermatic cord suspends the testis and consists of the testicular artery, deferential artery, cremasteric artery, pampiniform plexus of veins, nerves, lymphatics and the vas deferens.
- The spermatic cord passes from the scrotum through the inguinal canal to the abdomen.
- The appendix testis and appendix epididymis are both embryological remnants.
- The appendix testis is found toward the superior pole of the testis.
- The appendix epididymis is located on the head of the epididymis.

Testicular blood supply (Fig. 14.4)

- The right and left testicular arteries arise from the aorta just distal to the renal arteries, enter the spermatic cord at the external inguinal ring and supply most of the blood to the testes.
- The testicular arteries course along the anterior aspect of the testis, piercing the tunica albuginea.
- A branch of the testicular artery is the transmediastinal artery which is present in approximately 50% of testes.
- The transmediastinal artery is usually accompanied by a vein and courses through the mediastinum.
- Each pampiniform plexus continues as the testicular vein.
- The right testicular vein drains into the IVC and the left testicular vein into the left renal vein.

CLINICAL ASPECTS – ERECTILE DYSFUNCTION

- This includes conditions responsible for difficulty to attain or maintain an erection.
- It is preferable to the former description of impotence.

Normal flaccid penis (Fig. 14.5a)

- When the penis is flaccid, the helicine arteries and the sinusoids of the corpus cavernosa are constricted.
- High peripheral resistance causes low arterial blood flow to the penis.
- The emissary veins are not compressed and are dilated, with relative venous drainage greater than arterial inflow.

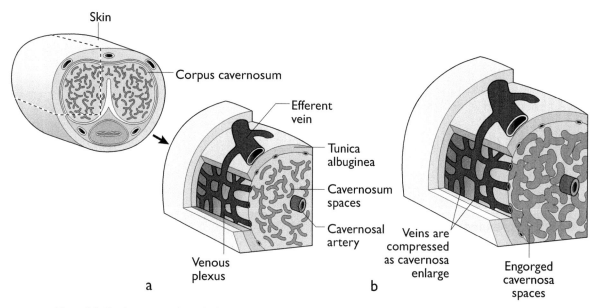

Fig. 14.5 *Anatomical and physiological changes associated with erection:*
a *Flaccid state.*
b *Erect state.*

Normal erection (Fig. 14.5b)

- Erection is a neurovascular phenomenon.
- Somatosensory afferents from the penis excite centers in the hindbrain and spinal cord.
- Sympathetic and parasympathetic autonomic efferent nerves then induce a vascular response.
- There is smooth muscle relaxation of helicine arteries resulting in vasodilation and increased arterial inflow.
- Distension of sinusoids of the corpus cavernosa causes mechanical compression of draining veins against the tunica albuginea, decreasing venous outflow. This is termed corporeal veno-occlusion.
- The combination of increased arterial flow and decreased venous outflow results in penile erection.

Etiology
Arterial insufficiency

- Aortic occlusion causing Leriche's syndrome (see Chapter 6).
- Common iliac or internal iliac artery stenosis.
- Diffuse internal pudendal or cavernosal artery stenosis or occlusion.
- It is a common cause in older patients, frequently associated with hypertension, diabetes, smoking and excessive alcohol consumption.

Venous leakage

- Insufficient corporeal veno-occlusion.
- Leakage through enlarged veins.
- This requires investigation as a possible cause in younger patients.

Neurogenic disorders
- Spinal cord injury.
- Surgical pelvic dissection, e.g. during repair of an abdominal aortic aneurysm.
- Sympathetic nerve block or sympathectomy.
- Multiple sclerosis.
- Autonomic nerve disorders.

Psychogenic disorders
- Depression.
- Social stress.
- Anxiety.

Clinical assessment
- Determine the nature of the sexual disorder and enquire about any psychiatric history.
- Obtain a medical history for diabetes, hypertension, heart disease, drug usage, hypercholesterolemia, alcohol ingestion and smoking.
- Examine the penis for physical deformities, tumors or trauma.

Treatment
- In the past, there were several options:
  - Penile intracavernosal injection of vasoactive drugs.
  - A penile prosthesis.
  - Arterial revascularization.
  - Surgery to ligate leaking veins.
- However, most patients are now treated with drugs such as Viagra.

CLINICAL ASPECTS – OTHER PENILE CONDITIONS

Etiology, pathology, clinical features and treatment
Peyronie's* disease
- This uncommon condition is probably due to repeated minor trauma.
- It is frequently associated with Dupuytren's contracture of the hands.
- Normal elastic tissue of the tunica albuginea is replaced by scar tissue, usually on the dorsum, leading to upward curvature during erection.
- Many patients have abnormal arterial studies.
- Treatment is conservative or by surgical correction.

Penile trauma
- This usually results from axial stress on the erect penis causing a tear of the tunica albuginea, rupture of the corpora cavernosa, and hemorrhage, referred to as a fractured penis. The rupture of the corpora cavernosa is generally transverse.
- Penile fracture most commonly occurs in the proximal or mid-shaft of the penis.
- Treatment usually requires surgical repair.

---

*François Gigot de La Peyronie, 1678–1747, French surgeon

High-flow priapism
- This is a persisting erection after trauma to the penis or perineum causes injury to an artery.
- There is high flow through a fistula from the cavernosal artery to the lacunae of the corpora cavernosa.
- Treatment usually requires surgical repair.

Low-flow priapism
- This is a persisting erection associated with decreased venous outflow.
- It is most frequently due to injection of vasoactive drugs to test for erectile dysfunction.
- It is treated conservatively.

CLINICAL ASPECTS – THE ACUTE SCROTUM
- Acute onset of scrotal pain with or without inflammation and swelling.
- Often seen in the emergency setting.

Torsion of the testis
Etiology and pathology
- It is usually associated with the 'bell-clapper' deformity – the tunica vaginalis has an abnormally high insertion on the spermatic cord and completely encircles the testis and epididymis leaving the testis free to rotate.
- The 'bell-clapper' deformity is usually bilateral.
- Torsion compromises venous then arterial, blood flow leading to testicular ischemia.
- The degree of torsion can range from 180° to 720° but complete occlusion of blood flow does not occur until about 450°.

Clinical features
- Torsion occurs most frequently in adolescent males.
- Presentation is with acute scrotal pain and swelling.
- The patient may also present with nausea, vomiting and low-grade fever.
- Intermittent acute pain suggests recurring partial torsion.

Treatment
- Urgent orchidopexy is required if the testis is viable, to untwist the testis and then fix it to the tunica vaginalis to prevent recurrence.
- Orchidectomy is performed if it is not viable.
- Orchidopexy for the non-affected side is indicated to prevent future torsion.

Torsion of testicular appendages
Etiology and pathology
- The appendages can twist if they have a narrow pedicle.
- This is more frequent than torsion of the testis.
- It usually occurs in males aged 7–14.
- The appendix testis is the most common appendage to undergo torsion.
- Calcification within the appendage may later result in 'scrotal pearls.'

Clinical features
- Torsion of either appendage produces pain similar to that experienced with testicular torsion.
- Torsion of a testicular appendage may be misinterpreted as testicular torsion or epididymo-orchitis.
- Reactive hydrocele and scrotal skin thickening may occur.

Treatment
- Conservative management is focused on pain relief which usually resolves with atrophy of the appendage.
- Surgical excision if pain persists or is too severe.

Epididymo-orchitis and epididymitis
Etiology and pathology
- This is due to bacterial infection, chemical inflammation caused by urine reflux through the spermatic cord or mechanical inflammation due to trauma.
- It is termed 'epididymitis' if only the epididymis is involved and 'epididymo-orchitis' if inflammation extends to the testis.
- In prepubertal males, it is almost always associated with a urinary tract anomaly.
- In adolescents and young adult males, it is often related to sexual activity and not to infection.
- In older males, it is usually due to prostatic obstruction causing stasis and secondary infection.

Clinical features
- The testis and epididymis or epididymis alone are enlarged.
- Examination of the urine will reveal or exclude bacterial infection.

Treatment
- If torsion is confidently excluded, then treatment is conservative with antibiotics if urinalysis shows infection.

PITFALL!
- It can be difficult to distinguish increased vascularity from an infection or a tumor.

Testicular trauma
Etiology
- Damage to the testis or epididymis can result from a direct blow or crush injury against the pubic bones.
- Injury may cause hemorrhage into the testis, hematocele or testicular rupture due to laceration of the tunica albuginea.

Clinical features
- Testicular trauma incurred during physical activities often causes severe pain of short duration.
- Pain that persists for more than one hour after trauma requires investigation to exclude testicular rupture or torsion.

● Pain that resolves promptly after trauma only to gradually recur suggests testicular injury.

Treatment
● Surgery is required for evacuate hematoma or repair rupture.
● Otherwise, if torsion is confidently excluded then treatment is conservative.

CLINICAL ASPECTS – OTHER SCROTAL DISORDERS

Varicocele
Etiology and pathology
● A varicocele is an abnormal enlargement of the pampiniform venous plexus which drains each testis.
● A primary varicocele occurs when venous dilation renders the valves of the testicular vein ineffective resulting in venous reflux and engorgement.
● A secondary varicocele results from venous compression by a renal carcinoma, other malignancies, retroperitoneal fibrosis or compression of the left renal vein by the superior mesenteric artery (SMA).

Clinical features
● They occur in young adult males with a prevalence of up to 20%.
● Most primary varicoceles occur on the left side, presumably due to drainage to the left renal vein at a right angle as opposed to the smoother drainage to the IVC on the right or due to left renal vein compression by the left testicular artery.
● However, they may be bilateral with the left side being larger.
● There may be no more than a palpable collection of veins while standing.
● Symptoms include dragging pain or a feeling of heaviness.
● Testicular atrophy occurs after a time, possibly causing impaired fertility.

Treatment
● Treatment is usually reserved for those with symptoms, testicular atrophy or infertility with a reduced semen count.
● Excision can be performed through an extraperitoneal abdominal, inguinal or scrotal approach.
● Closure can be affected by endovascular catheterization and embolization.

Testicular tumors
Pathology
● The most common testicular carcinomas are germ-cell tumors (95%).
● They are divided into two groups termed 'seminomas' and 'non-seminomas.'
● Seminomas are derived from seminiferous cells.
● Non-seminoma subtypes are teratoma, yolk-sac tumor and embryonal carcinoma.
● There can be mixed seminoma and non-seminoma cell tumors.
● Metastatic testicular lymphomas occur.
● Benign tumors derived from supportive and hormone-producing cells are termed 'stromal tumors' and include Sertoli's and Leydig's cell tumors.*

*Enrico Sertoli, 1842–1910, Italian pathologist
*Franz leydig, 1821–1908, German anatomist

- About 2–3% of males with prior testicular cancer later develop cancer in the other testis.
- Lymphatic metastasis can occur to para-aortic lymph nodes in the abdomen, mediastinum or cervical region.
- Systemic metastasis can occur to most organs.

Etiology
- Testicular cancers are most common in white men.
- Testicular cancers are considerably more common in undescended testes, which occur in 3% of young males, even after they have been surgically drawn down into the scrotum.
- Other factors implicated are family history, genetic disorders, Klinefelter's syndrome, mumps orchitis, cannabis smoking and HIV infection.

Clinical features
- Seminomas usually occur in males aged 20–40.
- Non-seminomas occur more frequently in males in their 20s.
- Symptoms include a painless hard swelling or lump in the testis, change in the size or shape of the testis or heaviness in the scrotum.
- Aching or pain in the lower abdomen, testis or scrotum.
- Enlargement or tenderness of breast tissue.

Modalities for diagnosis
- Duplex ultrasound.
- Blood tests for tumor markers.
- Computed tomography to locate metastases.
- Histological examination of the excised testis. Biopsy is avoided to prevent spread to the scrotum.

Differential diagnosis
- Epididymitis or epididymo-orchitis.
- Hematocele.
- Varicocele.

Treatment
- Treatment is by transinguinal orchidectomy.
- This is frequently supplemented by radiotherapy and/or chemotherapy according to the histology and spread of the tumor.
- Only one testis is required to maintain normal fertility and hormone production.
- Retroperitoneal lymph node dissection is now rarely performed.
- The cure rate is >90% if there are no metastases and 80% even with metastases.

Hydrocele, pyocele and hematocele
Etiology
- Pyoceles and hematoceles are rare.
- A hydrocele is a serous collection, a pyocele a purulent collection, and a hematocele a blood collection within the visceral and parietal layers of the tunica vaginalis.
- A hydrocele may be idiopathic or develop due to testicular torsion, trauma, infection or tumor.

- A pyocele is often associated with epididymo-orchitis or rupture of an intratesticular abscess.
- A hematocele is most commonly secondary to trauma, surgery or tumor.
- Fournier's* gangrene is a complication of a pyocele.

Clinical features
- A hydrocele may present as a painless scrotal swelling whereas a pyocele and a hematocele are painful.
- A hydrocele is a simple fluid collection around the anterolateral aspect of the testis.
- A pyocele and a hematocele are more complex lesions.

Treatment
- Treatment ranges from bed rest to surgical repair.

WHAT DOCTORS NEED TO KNOW

Erectile dysfunction
- Is there reduced arterial inflow?
- Is there venous leakage?
- Are there no vascular abnormalities, suggesting a psychological or neurological cause?
- Is there a cavernosal abnormality such as Peyronie's disease?
- Is there penile trauma?

The scrotum
- What is the cause of the presentation of acute scrotum?
- Is there torsion and if so is it testicular or of a testicular appendage?
- Is epididymitis or epididymo-orchitis present?
- Is a varicocele unilateral or bilateral?
- Is a varicocele associated with normal or reduced testicular size?
- Is a hydrocele, pyocele, or hematocele present?
- Is a testicular tumor present?

THE DUPLEX SCAN – PENILE STUDIES

Abbreviations
- Peak systolic velocity (cm/s) – PSV
- End-diastolic velocity (cm/s) – EDV
- Resistance index – RI = (PSV − EDV)/PSV
- Acceleration time – AT.

Indications for scanning
- Erectile dysfunction to detect impaired arterial inflow or venous leakage.
- To detect penile plaques in Peyronie's disease.
- Duplex flow characteristics as the preliminary investigation to diagnose the cause of priapism.
- Assessment of penile trauma.

*Jean Alfred Fournier, 1832–1914, French dermatologist

Normal findings
While the penis is flaccid
- The tunica albuginea is seen on B-mode as a linear hyperechoic sheath covering the corpora cavernosa.
- It is not possible to detect the helicine arteries even with power Doppler.
- There is low-resistance forward systolic and diastolic flow.
- The PSV in the cavernosal artery is >40 cm/s (Fig. 14.6).
- The EDV is 5–10 cm/s due to low intracavernosal resistance.

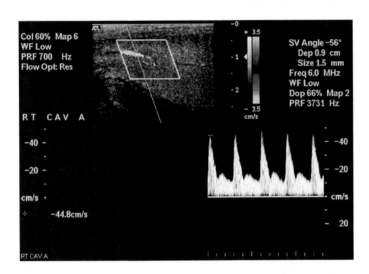

Fig. 14.6 *Normal spectral Doppler trace from a cavernosal artery in the flaccid penis.*

During erection
- Flow becomes apparent in the cavernosal and helicine arteries.
- There are progressive changes in diastolic flow:
  - In the early phase, there is prominent diastolic flow due to decreased resistance.
  - End-diastolic flow is then lost as intracavernosal pressure rises, increasing resistance.
  - Reverse end-diastolic flow is then seen as intracavernosal pressure exceeds the diastolic pressure.
  - Diastolic flow is lost when the penis becomes rigid.
- There is increased PSV >80 cm/s in the proximal cavernosal arteries.
- The cavernosal artery demonstrates a >70% increase in diameter.
- There is increased venous flow in the veins in the initial phase.
- Venous flow then falls and disappears with full rigidity.
- There is an increase in RI >0.90 to indicate sufficient venous occlusion.

Criteria for diagnosing erectile dysfunction
Arteriogenic
- In the flaccid penis, PSV <25–30 cm/s and AT >80 ms in the cavernosal arteries may be sufficient to make the diagnosis. This indicates extensive aortoiliac or pudendal arterial disease.
- During erection, arterial insufficiency is recognized by lack of dilation and the normal increase of PSV in the proximal cavernosal arteries; an abnormal result is defined as PSV <30 cm/s.

Venous leakage

- This is considered if the cavernosal arteries dilate and demonstrate PSV >25 cm/s, an EDV >5 cm/s and a reduction in the RI to <0.85.
- High EDV in the cavernosal arteries indicates low peripheral resistance to venous flow.
- Presence of venous flow at full rigidity.
- Ultrasound cannot provide an absolute diagnosis of venous leakage, so that it needs to be confirmed with cavernosometry or cavernosography.

Indications for Peyronie's disease

- On B-mode, thickening and an increased echogenicity of the tunica albuginea indicate fibrosis and calcification.

Indications for penile trauma

- On B-mode, a tunica albuginea tear can be visualized as an interruption of its thin echogenic line.
- On B-mode, a corpora cavernosa rupture can be identified as an irregular hyper- or hypoechoic collection in the corpora cavernosa.
- On B-mode, high-flow priapism will show as an irregular hypoechoic region in the corpora cavernosa after injury (Fig. 14.7). The lacunar spaces of the corpora cavernosa may be enlarged.
- On spectral Doppler, cavernosal artery flow will be normal or may increase with high-flow priapism.
- On color Doppler, the fistula will be identified by its false aneurysm-like shape with high velocities and turbulent flow (Fig. 14.8).

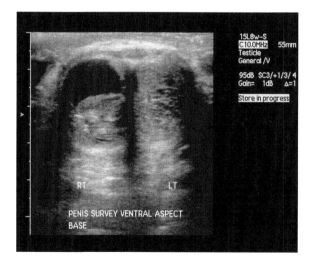

Fig. 14.7 *B-mode image of high-flow priapism.*
Image kindly supplied by Martin Necas, Hamilton, New Zealand.

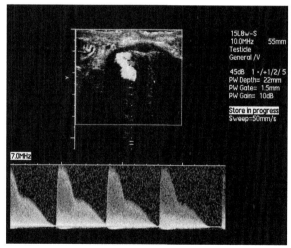

Fig. 14.8 *Color and spectral Doppler image of high-flow priapism.*
Image kindly supplied by Martin Necas, Hamilton, New Zealand.

THE DUPLEX SCAN – SCROTUM AND CONTENTS

Indications for scanning
- Acute testicular pain or swelling.
- Varicocele.

Normal findings
- The tunica albuginea is seen as a thin echogenic band around the testis.
- The space between the visceral and parietal layers of the tunica vaginalis is seen as a thin echolucent rim adjacent to the head of the epididymis. This should not be misinterpreted as a hydrocele.
- The mediastinum testis appears as an echogenic cord extending craniocaudal through the testis.
- The normal prepubertal testis has low- to medium-level echogenicity and is homogeneous.
- The normal pubertal and postpubertal testis has medium-level echogenicity and is homogeneous.
- The head of the epididymis is slightly more echogenic or is isoechoic to the normal testis. Its echotexture may be coarser. It has a length of 5–12 mm.
- The body of the epididymis is usually indistinguishable from the surrounding tissue and is 2–4 mm in diameter.
- The tail of the epididymis is seen as a curved structure inferior to the testis and is also 2–4 mm in diameter.
- The intratesticular arteries have generally low-resistance flow.
- The appendix testis and appendix epididymis are small and hyperechoic, and may be difficult to see if normal and easier to see if surrounded by hydrocele.
- The spermatic cord shows as multiple hypoechoic structures that are linear in the longitudinal plane and circular in the transverse plane.
- The normal diameter of pampiniform veins is 0.5–1.5 mm with no reflux.
- Normal scrotal wall thickness is 2–8 mm.

Indications for testicular torsion
- Highly pulsatile arterial flow with an absent diastolic component and may have a reduced PSV compared with the other testis (Figs 14.9 and 14.10).
- There is an absence of arterial flow in the twisted segment of the vessels.
- There is loss of phasicity with respiration in veins affected by torsion.
- The appearance depends on the duration of torsion.
- Within 6 hours, the testis and epididymis may be slightly enlarged.
- The testis and epididymis head may be more hypoechoic because of edema due to venous and lymphatic obstruction.
- After 24 hours, the testis will have a heterogeneous appearance due to vascular congestion, hemorrhage and infarction.
- Spiral twisting of the spermatic cord may be seen with color Doppler.
- The spermatic cord below the torsion may appear as a round or oval extratesticular homogeneous mass.
- Normal testicular echogenicity and lack of scrotal wall thickening or reactive hydrocele is a strong predictor that the testis is viable.
- After 24 hours, echogenicity of the testis becomes heterogeneous, a sign that it is no longer viable.
- The presence of flow does not exclude torsion.

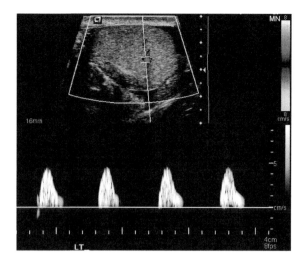

Fig. 14.9 *Spectral Doppler image of flow within testicle in torsion.*

Image kindly supplied by Martin Necas, Hamilton, New Zealand.

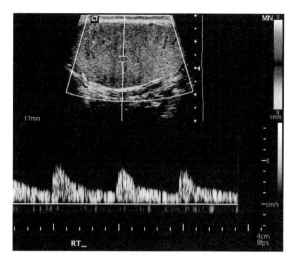

Fig. 14.10 *Spectral Doppler image of flow within normal testicle.*

Image kindly supplied by Martin Necas, Hamilton, New Zealand.

Indications for torsion of testicular appendages

- B-mode shows a hyperechoic mass with a central hypoechoic area adjacent to the testis or epididymis.
- B-mode may show testicular edema and epididymal enlargement.
- Color Doppler ultrasound demonstrates increased blood flow around the testicular appendages.
- No color flow is demonstrated in normal testicular appendages and those that have undergone torsion.
- Color Doppler ultrasound shows that blood flow within the testis is normal.
- A 'scrotal pearl' will be demonstrated on B-mode as a calcified stone within an echolucent hydrocele (Fig. 14.11).

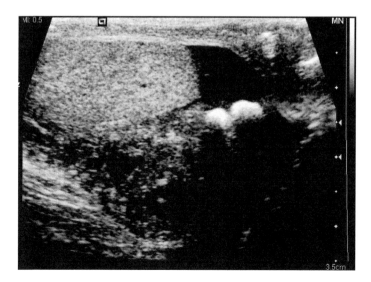

Fig. 14.11 *B-mode image of 'scrotal pearl.'*

Image kindly supplied by Martin Necas, Hamilton, New Zealand.

Indications for epididymitis and epididymo-orchitis

- B-mode findings are of an enlarged hyper- or hypoechoic epididymis for epididymitis.
- Color Doppler will demonstrate increased blood flow in and around the epididymis.
- B-mode will show testicular involvement as well as epididymo-orchitis.
- Color and power Doppler ultrasound will show increased blood flow in and around the testis as well (Fig. 14.12).
- B-mode will show edema of the testis with diffuse or local heterogeneous echogenicity.
- In the chronic condition, multiple hypoechoic lesions may be seen within the testicular parenchyma.
- B-mode may demonstrate a hydrocele or pyocele with scrotal wall thickening.
- Arterial flow will have a low peripheral resistance and a relatively high end-diastolic velocity.

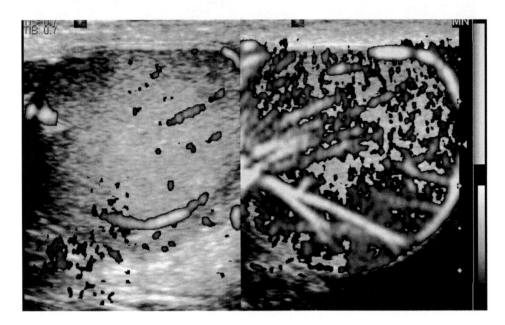

Fig. 14.12 *Power Doppler image of increased blood flow with epididymo-orchitis (right) compared with normal testicle (left).*

Image kindly supplied by Martin Necas, Hamilton, New Zealand.

Indications for testicular rupture

- B-mode can demonstrate testicular rupture by an interruption of the tunica albuginea, scrotal wall thickening, a large hematocele, hematoma in the testis or a heterogeneous testis with an irregular border.
- Color and power Doppler can demonstrate focal areas of absent flow.

Indications of varicocele

- Varicocele is defined by dilation of the small vessels of the pampiniform plexus to >2 mm diameter (Fig. 14.13).
- A Valsalva maneuver or standing will show reflux with color and spectral Doppler (Fig. 14.14).

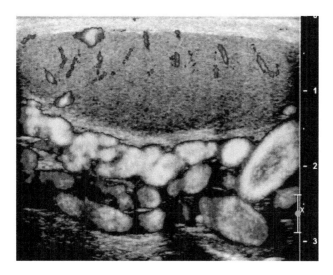

Fig. 14.13 *Power Doppler image of a varicocele.*

Image kindly supplied by Martin Necas, Hamilton, New Zealand.

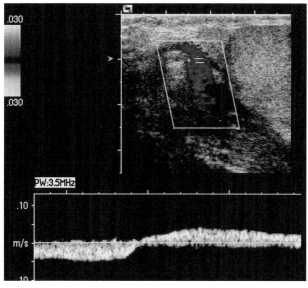

Fig. 14.14 *Spectral Doppler of reflux within a varicocele.*

Image kindly supplied by Martin Necas, Hamilton, New Zealand.

Indications for testicular tumors

- B-mode determines the location, size and characteristics of the tumor such as cystic or solid, uniform or heterogeneous or sharply circumscribed or poorly defined.
- Pure seminomas are typically homogeneous and hypoechoic without calcification. Occasionally a seminoma is more heterogeneous, rarely with necrosis.
- Non-seminoma germ-cell tumors tend to be much more heterogeneous and frequently contain cystic areas and coarse calcification.
- Stromal tumors are usually homogeneous and hypoechoic and are often multiple and bilateral. Larger tumors may become more heterogeneous due to hemorrhage and necrosis.
- Testicular lymphoma metastases appear similar to primary tumors.
- Most testicular tumors show flow with color, spectral and power Doppler but these do not help to differentiate between various tumors.

Indications for hydrocele, hematocele and pyocele
- B-mode will show anechoic fluid surrounding the anterolateral aspect of the testis with hydrocele.
- B-mode will show an echo-filled lesion around the testis with hematocele and pyocele.

PROTOCOLS FOR SCANNING

Prepare the patient
- The investigation is very sensitive and usually best performed by a male sonographer.
- If a vasoactive drug is to be administered, written consent must be obtained from the patient for the examination and possible side effects.
- A doctor will be present if provocative tests are performed to produce an erection.
- For penile studies, maintain a serious attitude.
- For scrotal studies, provide reassurance and adequate analgesia.

Position the patient and select windows
- For most studies, place the patient supine with the penis placed dorsally on the pubic region (erection position).
- Rolled towels on either side may help to stabilize the penis.
- For scrotal studies, lift the penis and cover it with a towel. With the legs slightly spread apart, support the scrotum with a towel rolled between the thighs.
- Use warm gel to prevent scrotal contraction.
- Stand the patient for a study for varicocele.
- For penile studies, place the transducer on the corpus cavernosa near the base of the penis from an anterolateral approach.
- Image the scrotum in transverse from the top of the scrotum.

Select the best transducer
- The penis, scrotum and scrotal vessels are examined with a high-frequency linear array transducer.
- For penile studies, use a low-frequency curved- or phased-array transducer to examine the aorta and iliac arteries (see Chapter 6).

Machine settings
- Set the wall filter and pulse repetition frequency (PRF) as low as possible.
- Adjust the color gain to display slow flow.
- Use a small, straight color sample box.
- Use power Doppler for low-flow states such as intratesticular flow with acute scrotum studies that cannot be detected by color Doppler.
- With scrotal studies, scan the asymptomatic testis first to set the ultrasound machine settings.

Scan the aorta, CIA and IIA
- Use B-mode and color and spectral Doppler to examine the aorta and each CIA and IIA. If present, calculate the severity of stenosis or extent of occlusion (see Chapter 6).

Scan the penis

- Begin at the base of the flaccid penis.
- In transverse B-mode, examine the corpora cavernosa and tunica albuginea and note their echogenicity and echotexture.
- Use color power and spectral Doppler to interrogate areas of hypogenicity for flow.
- In B-mode, examine the tunica albuginea for a tear.
- In color Doppler and longitudinal, angle the transducer medially to identify the cavernosal arteries.
- In B-mode, measure the diameter of each cavernosal artery.
- Record a spectral trace and note the PSV and EDV in both cavernosal arteries.
- Note the RI of the cavernosal arteries.
- If a vasoactive substance is given, the doctor will assess the clinical response. The cavernosal arteries are then examined as above at 4–5 min post-injection and at 2- to 3-min intervals until full erection.
- With color, power and spectral Doppler, examine for venous flow at full rigidity.

Scan the scrotum and contents

- Scan the unaffected side first to familiarize the patient with the procedure and to give a baseline for anatomy and flow.
- Scan the scrotum and contents in longitudinal and transverse.
- Use B-mode to examine the echogenicity and echotexture and measure the size of each testis and epididymis compared with the contralateral side.
- Use B-mode to examine for suspected tumor; measure the size and note the location and B-mode characteristics.
- Use color, power and spectral Doppler to examine for intratesticular, epididymal and suspected lesion flow.
- The epididymis is best scanned in longitudinal.
- Use B-mode to examine for fluid in the layers of the tunica vaginalis. Note whether the fluid is echolucent or contains echoes.
- The testicular artery and pampiniform plexus can be identified within the spermatic cord. Examine the arteries and veins at the level of the inguinal canal.
- Use color and spectral Doppler to confirm absence of flow in twisted vessels and loss of intratesticular flow with testicular torsion. Note loss of phasicity of flow in veins.
- Use B-mode to examine for torsion of testicular appendages or 'scrotal pearls.'
- Use color Doppler to examine for absent blood flow in the appendage and increased adjacent flow.
- Use B mode to examine the tunica albuginea for rupture.
- If a varicocele is suspected, in B-mode measure maximum diameters of the pampiniform plexus in longitudinal and transverse.
- Take spectral traces within the pampiniform plexus to demonstrate reflux, with the patient breathing normally and performing the Valsalva maneuver or standing.
- Use B-mode to measure scrotal wall thickness.

ULTRASOUND IMAGES TO RECORD

Penile

- Sample spectral traces of the aorta and each CIA and IIA.
- Spectral traces proximal to, at and distal to each aortoiliac stenosis. Note the location from an anatomical landmark, the extent and the severity.
- Spectral trace proximal to, distal to and within aortoiliac occlusions. Note the location from an anatomical landmark and the extent.
- Transverse B-mode image of corpora cavernosum.
- Transverse B-mode image of tunica albuginea.
- B-mode diameters of cavernosal arteries pre- and post-stimulation.
- Sample spectral traces and note the RI of cavernosal arteries pre- and post-stimulation.
- Color and power Doppler and sample spectral traces of venous flow pre- and post-stimulation.

Scrotal

- In transverse, B-mode and color and power Doppler dual images comparing the same portion of each testis.
- B-mode diameter of each testis and length of each epididymis.
- B-mode images of tunica vaginalis; note presence of echoes within fluid.
- B-mode images of tunica albuginea.
- Sample spectral trace in each testicular artery.
- Sample spectral traces with the patient supine, standing and with the Valsalva maneuver in pampiniform venous plexus.
- B-mode diameter of veins of the pampiniform plexus.
- B-mode images of tumor; measure the size and note the location and B-mode characteristics.
- Color Doppler images of flow in tumor.
- B-mode and color Doppler images of torsion of testicular appendages or 'scrotal pearls'.
- B-mode measurement of scrotal thickness.

WORKSHEET

- Note the information about images from ultrasound images to record.

15 ULTRASOUND-GUIDED INTERVENTIONS

Ultrasound techniques are available to guide interventions for arterial and venous disease. The following is not an exhaustive list.

ENDOVASCULAR TREATMENT OF OCCLUSIVE ARTERIAL DISEASE

- It is traditional to perform balloon dilatation or stenting under fluoroscopic control in a radiology suite.
- However, these procedures can be performed with a combination of B-mode to show passage of guidewires, catheters and balloons, and color and spectral Doppler to identify stenosis or occlusion and confirm that it has been restored toward normal by treatment.
- This is best suited to the accessible femoropopliteal arterial segment.

TREATMENT OF FALSE ANEURYSMS

- False aneurysms now most often result from arterial puncture and insertion of a sheath in the common femoral artery during peripheral or coronary angiography, or cardiac endovascular treatment.
- Conservative ultrasound-guided techniques can permanently occlude the aneurysm to avoid open surgical repair.
- False aneurysms <2 cm can be treated with compression therapy.
- Larger false aneurysms can be occluded by thrombin injection using ultrasound guidance.
- Patients with a false aneurysm with a wide 'neck' should be treated surgically because the risk of an arterial occlusion after thrombin injection cannot be excluded.

Ultrasound-guided compression
- Pressure is applied at a strategic point to occlude the connection from artery to aneurysm so that stasis within the aneurysm causes it to thrombose.
- This is effective in >75%, but the process frequently needs to be repeated and each session can take up to 60 min so it is very taxing for the patient and sonographer.
- Success is less likely if the neck is wide or the aneurysm large or long-standing, if there is considerable pain making it difficult to maintain compression or if the patient is anticoagulated.

Ultrasound-guided thrombin injection
- This is an attractive alternative to compression.
- However, local arterial or venous thrombosis and pulmonary embolism have been reported as complications.
- Under local anesthesia, a 20-gauge needle is placed in the aneurysm well away from the neck and human thrombin is injected slowly until the aneurysm occludes.

- Color Doppler and B-mode scanning show the process well (Fig. 15.1).
- The aneurysm is almost always permanently controlled within a few minutes at the first treatment, even in anticoagulated patients.

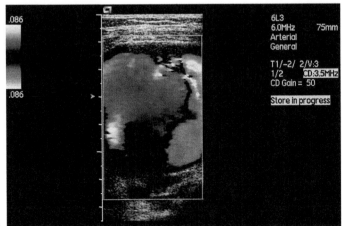

a

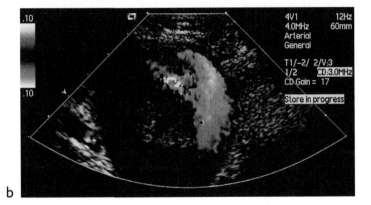

b

Fig. 15.1 *Color Doppler image of ultrasound-guided thrombin injection of false aneurysm:*
a *Partial thrombosis of false aneurysm.*
b *Increase of thrombosis with time.*

Images kindly supplied by Martin Necas, Hamilton, New Zealand.

TREATMENT OF CHRONIC VENOUS DISEASE

Ultrasound-guided sclerotherapy

- Traditional treatment for varicose veins by surgical ligation and stripping has been supplemented in recent years by ultrasound-guided sclerotherapy (UGS) of the saphenous trunk or tributaries.
- Planning treatment requires a careful preoperative venous duplex study (see Chapter 11).
- The sclerosant can be used as a liquid or foam.
- Hold the transducer exactly perpendicular to the skin to show the vein in longitudinal to guide the needle.
- Place the needle exactly in the midline of the transducer axis to show both its full length and sclerosant in the vein as it is injected (Fig. 15.2).
- Alternately, hold the transducer to show the vein in transverse and approach with the needle from one or other side.
- This allows the transducer to be shifted up or down to bring the needle into view if it has not been placed correctly, but it does not show any length of the vein.

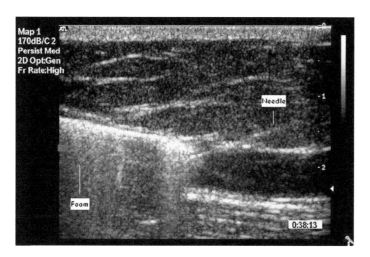

Fig. 15.2 *B-mode image of foamed sclerosant being injected into the great saphenous vein during ultrasound-guided sclerotherapy.*

Ultrasound-guided endovenous laser ablation or radiofrequency closure

● These two techniques are favored by most phlebologists for larger-diameter saphenous veins.

● The vein is punctured as far distally as possible with an angiogram needle.

● Guided by B-mode, a guidewire is passed to the saphenous junction and a long sheath is passed over the wire to just below the junction (Fig. 15.3).

● Local anesthetic is then injected into the saphenous sheath around the vein along its full length using B-mode guidance (Fig. 15.4).

● The guidewire is removed and replaced with either a laser probe or a radiofrequency probe.

● This is passed along the vein to just below the saphenous junction and the position of the probe tip is confirmed by B-mode.

● The entire length from below the saphenous junction to the puncture site is destroyed as the activated probe is withdrawn.

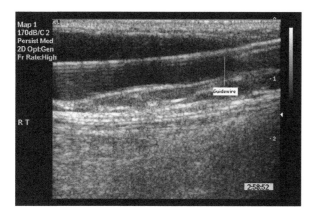

Fig. 15.3 *B-mode image of a guidewire inserted into the great saphenous vein during ultrasound-guided endovenous laser ablation.*

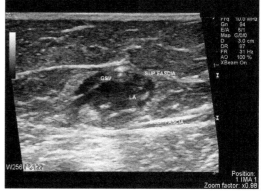

Fig. 15.4 *Transverse B-mode image of injection of local anesthetic into the perivenous saphenous sheath during endovenous laser ablation.*

Mechanical ablation

- A technique is now available to destroy the venous intima by causing mechanical damage together with infusion of a sclerosant drug.
- The probe is passed up the vein after puncture just as for thermal ablation.
- However, tumescent anesthesia is not required because the procedure is essentially painless.
- The probe has a floppy wire at the tip, which when activated by a motor thrashes around within the lumen causing intimal damage. The sclerosant is an added measure for intimal destruction.
- The probe is slowly withdrawn as sclerosant is slowly injected.

NEEDLE PUNCTURE

- Conventional ultrasound can be used to guide a vascular puncture for angiography or endovascular intervention.
- This can shorten the time taken and increase success rates, particularly for difficult cases with disease at the puncture site or obesity.
- Needles with an ultrasound crystal at the tip have been used.

CENTRAL VENOUS ACCESS

- A *central venous catheter* is inserted through the internal jugular, subclavian, axillary or femoral veins.
- A *peripherally inserted central catheter (PICC line)* is inserted through a peripheral vein such as the cephalic, basilic, median cubital or brachial veins.
- The catheter's tip rests in the superior vena cava or right atrium, preferably at the cavoatrial junction.
- They can be left in place for long periods of time.

Types of catheters
Non-tunneled central venous catheters
- These protrude through the skin at the site of insertion in the neck or groin.
- They have a greater risk of infection or accidental displacement.

Tunneled central venous catheters
- These are tunneled under the skin from the insertion site to a separate exit site, for example on the chest.
- The access ports for the catheter and its attachments are less visible than if they were to directly protrude from the neck.
- Separation of the insertion and exit sites reduces the risk of infection and provides a more secure fixation.
- A commonly used tunneled catheter is the Hickman catheter.*
- Another type is the Permacath, commonly used for short-term hemodialysis.

Implanted central venous ports (Portacath)
- A port is similar to a tunneled catheter but is left entirely under the skin.
- There may be a small reservoir for containing injected medications.

---

*Dr Robert Hickman, pediatric nephrologist, Seattle, USA

- An implanted port is less obvious than a tunneled catheter and requires minimal care.
- The port is accessed by special needles.
- It is best suited to patients who require less frequent access over a long period.

PICC line

- This is the simplest catheter to insert and remove.
- It is the most suitable for short-term use.
- It has less risk of complications during insertion.
- It has less risk of causing serious infection.
- It can be more readily repeated.
- It is more difficult to conceal.

Insertion of a central venous catheter and PICC line

- They are inserted under sterile conditions.
- The vein is located with B-mode ultrasound.
- The vein is punctured with a needle under ultrasound guidance, confirmed by aspirating venous blood.
- A guidewire is passed through the needle which is then removed.
- A dilator is passed over the guidewire to enlarge the tract.
- The catheter is advanced over the guidewire to the distal superior vena cava, cavoatrial junction or right atrium, and the guidewire is removed.
- A PICC line may have a single or multiple lumina.
- Central venous lines have multiple lumina.
- All lumina of the catheter are aspirated to ensure that the catheter is positioned inside the vein and then flushed.
- There is a cuff under the exit site for a tunneled central venous catheter to help prevent dislodgement.
- The catheter is fixed at the exit site with sutures or staples.
- The inserted portion of a PICC line varies from 25 cm to 60 cm in length.
- Some PICC lines can be trimmed to the required length before insertion whereas others are inserted to the required length with the excess left outside.
- A chest radiograph is performed to confirm the correct position and that no pneumothorax has occurred with subclavian or internal jugular vein puncture.

Indications for central venous catheters or PICC lines

- Long-term intravenous administration of antibiotics, pain medications or chemotherapy.
- Long-term parenteral nutrition.
- Intravenous therapy when peripheral venous access not possible.
- Administration of drugs that would cause peripheral phlebitis.
- Plasmapheresis.
- Short-term hemodialysis.
- Repetitive blood sampling.
- Monitoring of central venous pressure.

Complications of central venous catheters or PICC lines
Complications during insertion

- Pneumothorax (subclavian or internal jugular vein puncture).
- Damage to an adjacent artery or nerve.

- Hemorrhage or hematoma.
- Air embolism.
- Malpositioning.
- Guidewire entrapment.
- Catheter transection or migration.
- Arrhythmias.

Late complications
- Systemic infection.
- Thrombosis of the axillary or subclavian veins (Fig. 15.5).
- Pinching of a catheter at the thoracic outlet.

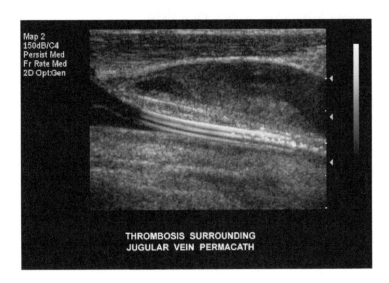

Fig. 15.5 B-mode image of thrombus around an intravenous catheter.

INTRAVASCULAR ULTRASOUND

- The technology is rapidly improving, currently with fine 3.5 French (Fr) catheters and high-frequency 20-MHz transducers available for B-mode and color Doppler imaging.
- Intravascular ultrasound (IVUS) is being increasingly used for peripheral arterial or venous and coronary arterial interventions to show the vessel lumen and wall, branches and tributaries and surrounding structures.
- This avoids radiation and contrast toxicity resulting from conventional fluoroscopic control.
- IVUS requires additional equipment and personnel and the expense of disposable probes, but it can be cost-effective.

During intervention for stenotic or occlusive arterial disease
- Benefits include the following:
  - Demonstrates complex anatomy and clarifies findings from arteriography.
  - Determines whether plaque is non-calcified or calcified and eccentric or concentric.
  - Accurately measures arterial diameters and extent of disease to select proper angioplasty balloon size.
  - Shows residual flaps or thrombus after endarterectomy.
  - Detects arterial rupture, intimal flaps or dissection after balloon dilation.

○ Confirms full expansion and attachment to the arterial wall for an endovascular stent or stent graft.

○ Can be used after surgery to detect late recurrent disease due to atherosclerosis or neointimal hyperplasia.

For endovascular aneurysm repair

● Intraoperative IVUS accurately measures aortic diameters to select the best-sized stent-graft; this helps to reduce the frequency of Type I endoleaks (see Chapter 6).

● It alters selection of graft size in approximately one-third of patients where size was calculated from a preoperative CT scan.

● It can assess outcome without completion arteriography to ensure that renal or suprarenal artery orifices have not been covered and to detect potential endoleaks.

● It can be used with other imaging modalities after initial stabilization to stage aortic dissections.

● It helps to guide placement of a stent-graft for aortic dissection and to select the site for fenestration to restore distal perfusion.

For diagnosis and endovascular treatment for vena cava or iliac vein compression

● IVUS is used to diagnose the cause of extrinsic major venous compression or intrinsic venous stenosis and associated thrombosis.

● It can be used to direct guidewire placement and endovascular treatment by balloon dilatation or stenting.

For IVC filter placement

● IVUS can be used to guide insertion of an inferior vena cava (IVC) filter in the intensive care unit.

● A single groin puncture is used for both IVUS and filter placement.

● Major branch veins, thrombosis, caval diameter and the ideal site for filter location are demonstrated without the need for contrast agents.

Index

Printed and bound by CPI Group (UK) Ltd, Croydon, CR0 4YY

23/10/2024

01777680-0007